Thalamus and its Cortex

Notes from a Seminar

Thalamus and its Cortex

Notes from a Seminar

Edison K. Miyawaki, M.D.

To order additional copies of this book, contact:
Xlibris
844-714-8691
www.Xlibris.com
Orders@Xlibris.com
825571

CONTENTS

In normal psychical life, sight-sensations do not make their appearance alone, but are accompanied by other sensations. We do not see optical images in an optical space, but we perceive the bodies round about us with their many and varied sensible qualities. Deliberate analysis is needed to single out the sight-sensations from these complexes. But even the total perceptions themselves are almost invariably accompanied by thoughts, wishes, and impulses. By sensations are excited, in animals, the movements of adaptation demanded by their conditions of life. If these conditions are simple, altering but little and slowly, immediate sensory excitation is sufficient. But the case is different where the conditions of life are intricate and variable. Here so simple a mechanism of adaptation cannot develop, still less would it lead to the accomplishment of the required ends.

–Ernst Mach (1914)

1

Preface: July, 2020

I fear that teaching at my medical school has changed, perhaps for the long-term future. A new academic year began this month. Our classes are now virtual.

Aren't there types of virtual learning *not* having to do images on a screen? In the current vernacular, "virtual" means something to the effect of "not in person." But one could resurrect a dictionary's definition of *virtual*–that which results *in essence*, though not in actual fact or form.

Not long ago, I envisioned a new seminar in which people responded to a reading list that I've compiled in books written over several years.[1] I had hoped that participants might talk to each other in light of a few good papers, most of them anatomical in nature. Now, however, I virtualize out of necessity, due to the circumstances of our time. I'll create my seminar *in essence*.

---

[1]   Prior monographs most pertinent to what follows are: *Teaching Hippocampal Anatomy* (2019), *The Visual Cortices* (2020), and *Beneath the Cortical Surface* (2020), all published by Xlibris (Bloomington, IN).

The participants address the relationship between thalamus and cortex. As you'll see, their observations, which I've collected into one place here, aren't trivial.

*

As the seminar's organizer and secretary, errors of commission and omission in what follows are my responsibility.

PART I

2

First Participant: His Categories of Sensation

An unlikely presence in a seminar on the brain, F.A.H. graduated from law school, but had studied neuroanatomy in his teens and early twenties, with particular attention to sensory systems. In a statement regarding why he wanted to participate, he wrote that "the fascination of physiological psychology never quite left me" (quoted in Birner, 1999). He was too interesting not to include among the participants.

*

One shouldn't self-congratulate, but it seemed as if F.A.H. had absorbed ideas in chapters entitled "Labeled Line" in *Beneath the Cortical Surface* and "A Note on Geniculocalcarine and Corticogeniculate" in *The Visual Cortices*.

Signals pass through wires, he observed, apologizing for the reductionist statement. But then he extended his simplification to envision a telephone exchange in which a wire or more than one wire connects/connect to a specific "bell." "All the wires connected with any one bell would then carry signals belonging to the same class" (Hayek, 1976a).[2]

F.A.H. acknowledged that a telephone exchange–a dated metaphor, to be sure, he said–didn't do justice to the brain's anatomy:

> The cerebral cortex is the highest and most complex of several 'bridges' which connect the afferent fibres conducting impulses from the peripheral receptors, and the efferent fibres conducting impulses to the motor organs. We must thus conceive of the central nervous system (and probably also of the cortex itself) as a hierarchy consisting of many superimposed levels of connexions, all of which may be concerned in the transmission of impulses from the afferent (sensory) to the efferent (motor) fibres. This conception of a hierarchy of centres or levels does, of course, not imply that these levels can always be sharply separated, either structurally or functionally, or that they are superimposed upon each other in a simple linear order (Hayek, 1976b).

He added that for all his interest in matters of the brain, "I never had a live teacher in psychology" (quoted in Ebenstein, 2003). Perhaps virtual learning, which is the absence of live teaching and classmates in a shared room, isn't to be underestimated. F.A.H. himself sounded like a dour, but inexplicably beloved teacher when he said things like "we must thus conceive."

---

[2]   There's subtlety to the nerve fiber-wire association, as Helmholtz discussed in the late 19th century: (please do read this passage to the very end, where there's a surprise) "The nerve fibres have been often compared with telegraphic wires traversing a country . . .. In the network of telegraphs that we find everywhere the same copper or iron wires carrying the same kind of movement, a stream of electricity, but producing the most different results in the various stations according to the auxiliary apparatus with which they are connected. At one station the effect is the ringing of a bell, at another a signal is moved, and at a third a recording instrument is set to work. . . . When the Atlantic cable was being laid, Sir William Thomson found that the slightest signals could be recognised by the sense of taste, if the wire was laid upon the tongue (Helmholtz, 1881, p. 205)."

The seminar's participants liked how suggestive he could be. Take the wire(s) and the bell: if there were many wires leading to one bell, then, in terms of the operation of the exchange, there's a bell that rings as a function of one or more afferents. There could be many connections and even (as in the case of internet telecommunication) hierarchies of connections, but there's only one bell.

To drive his point home, F.A.H. proposed a thought experiment in which we envision a machine that separates balls–the balls, not bells, differing only in their diameters–into two receptacles:

> . . . the machine will always place the balls with a diameter of 16, 18, 28, 31, 32, and 40 mm in a receptacle marked *A*, the balls with a diameter of 17, 22, 30, and 35 in a receptacle marked *B*, and so forth. The balls placed by the machine into the same receptacle will then be said to belong to the same class, and the balls placed by it into different receptacles to belong to so many different classes. The fact that a ball is placed by the machine into a particular receptacle thus forms the sole criterion for assigning it to a particular class (Hayek, 1976a).

P.G-R., a participant whom we'll introduce in the next chapter, expressed mystification about the purpose of such a machine, since, by its design, it didn't help to determine whether a 35 mm ball was larger than the 30 mm ball or, for that matter, whether a 16 mm ball was smaller than a 17 mm ball. "This machine doesn't really measure," she offered as she adjusted her glasses.

Unfazed, F.A.H. continued that sensation had to be a function of categories, like receptacles *A* and *B*, *and* that categorization of some type must be happening in what he previously termed the "hierarchy of centres or levels." Why "must"?

F.A.H. reminded us of numbers relevant to brains: nerve cells within cortex far exceed the number of afferent fibres to them–ten thousand million neurons as opposed to a few million afferent fibres (Hayek, 1976b). The orders-of-magnitude difference must mean something in terms of function of the whole.

His ball-sorting machine was an artifice in light of which two issues arise, he said. The first is how an afferent impulse is classified–worked over, one could say—by the broad swath of cortex. The second is whether there really is a correspondence between a ball's actual size and attributes of the sensory category into which a ball is placed.

We started to think about F.A.H.'s machine in relationship to neuroanatomy, but . . . let's pause for decorum first. The seminar's participants should be introduced before describing the group's work.

3

The Others

There was J.VN., who, as the clinical phrase goes, appeared older than stated age, because he wore dark, banker's suits and narrow neckties to all our sessions. His background was somehow very mathematical–"somehow," because his forte, he said, was applied, not exactly pure, mathematics related to such things as weather, gambling games, eddies of force in munitions explosions, and computers. Like everyone else in the group, he was smart–much more so than the seminar's organizer. Indeed all the participants whom I selected were unnecessarily smart. J.VN. was quirky; I liked him.

There was P.G.-R., a Vassar grad and the only woman in our group. How to capture her in a sentence? As was evident in her application, she had read all the monographs in the series serving as the basis of the seminar. She said of *The Visual Cortices* (I'll paraphrase her[3]): As interesting and influential as visual system research surely is, I'm not attracted to it. How could a person not like her?

Last of the four was R.W.G., who had more than a thought or two about thalamocortex, based on his background in physiology.

---

[3]   I use a quotation cited at: vcencyclopedia.vassar.edu/alumni/patricia-goldman-rakic.html[.]

4

Series and Sensation

J.VN. wondered if it mattered to the machine's operation whether a 17-mm ball was presented to it *before* an 18-mm ball. It shouldn't matter, he thought. But there are implications if, on the one hand, the order of the balls was irrelevant and, on the other, if the order was very relevant. You see, he continued,

> . . . parallel and serial operation are not unrestrictedly substitutable for each other . . .. More specifically, not everything serial can be immediately paralleled–certain operations can only be performed after certain others, and not simultaneously with them (i.e., they must use the results of the latter). In such a case, the transition from a serial scheme to a parallel one may be impossible, or it may be possible but only concurrently with a change in the logical approach and organization of the procedure. Conversely, the desire to serialize a parallel procedure may impose new requirements . . .. Specifically, it will almost always create new memory requirements, since the results of the operations that are performed first must be stored while the operations that come after these are performed (Von Neumann, 2000).

In a process having only to do with inclusion into either category *A* or *B*, the temporal order of different sized balls presented to the machine is immaterial. The machine doesn't have to remember the order of presentation, because only the categories matter. And it doesn't need to have a memory-storage component to its design—no memory needed, that is, of its prior operations. Is all the above consistent, J.V.N. asked, with how the brain *senses*?

R.W.G. pounced:

> . . . messages carried to the brain from the eye, the ear, the muscle receptors, the skin, etc. function to inform the central sensory pathways about events impinging on peripheral receptors. That is, they *represent* external events. . . . [S]uch a view, while clearly in accord with known relationships between sensory events and neural activity in ascending pathways to cortex, ignores the fact that the neural activity reaching cortex represents more than merely the information about events that impinge on peripheral receptors. . . . [A]fferents to the thalamus are commonly made up of branching axons that send one branch to the thalamus for transfer to cortex and another branch to motor or premotor centers for a role in action. . . . [These branched axons provide] the cortex with information about the instructions that have already been sent to the motor centers (Guillery, 2005).

P.G-R. thought that how the brain afferents (informs) itself was worth the group's attention. As R.W.G. observes, the thalamus must play a role, she said.

*

The quasi-fictional seminar described in the preceding pages outlines two topics of interest, aside from all the anatomy that follows in this monograph.

Regarding our participants, alas, all four have passed: Friedrich A. Hayek (F.A.H.) in 1992, John von Neumann (J.V.N.) in 1957, Patricia Goldman-Rakic (P.G.-R.) in 2003, and R.W. Guillery (R.W.G.) in 2017.

I chose these luminaries no longer with us for their perspectives on two questions:

1. What does "category" have to do with sensation?

2. It's not hard to find evidence for both serial and parallel processing in a brain. Think about the visual pathway from retina to thalamus, then visual cortical processing along "what" and "where" streams (see *The Visual Cortices*). But what's the role of memory in sensation?

PART II

5

Just Looking at Lateral
Geniculate Nuclei

Let's visualize the nuclei in question. I won't label this image, because it's better to describe in words than to point without looking carefully:

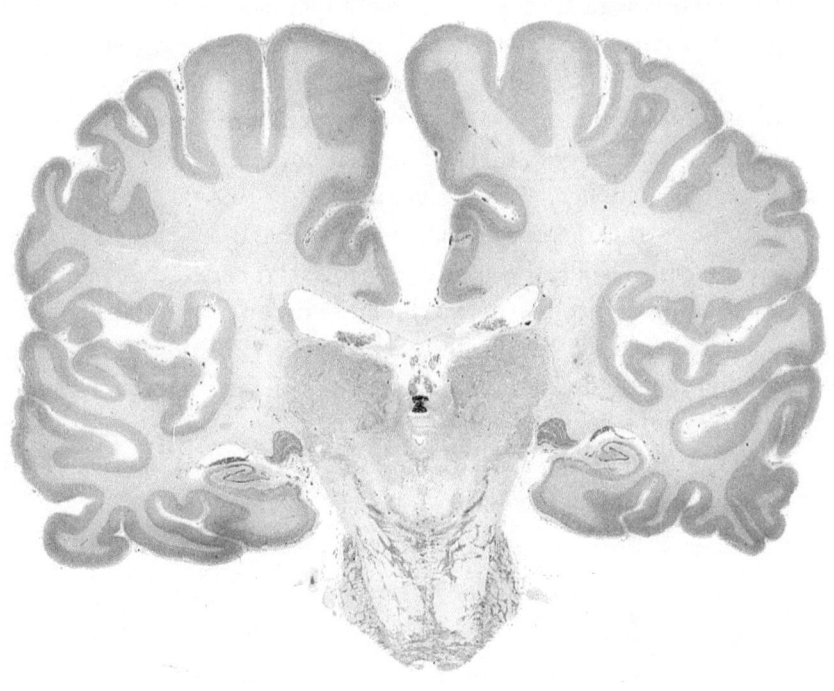

The stain darkens cells; white matter remains white.
This chapter addresses just what we see in the image.

*

Lateral geniculate nucleus (henceforward, LGN) differs from other locales in thalamus, because of its dark staining, both in the parvo- (dorsally located) and magno- (ventrally located) cellular layers, and because of its overt lamination.

There are six layers of neurons in a human LGN (in other primates, there are fewer layers; the owl monkey LGN, for example, has four). But much depends on what part of human LGN you examine: anteriorly and posteriorly (in rostral LGN and caudal LGN), the dorsally-located laminae of LGN *always* fuse to a degree, lending the impression of fewer than six layers (Jones, 1985a).

*

One should be careful when mentioning "dorsal LGN," because the two LGNs that we see in the image *belong completely to* dorsal thalamus, in the strict embryological sense of "dorsal thalamus." There's also a ventral LGN, part of ventral thalamus, which receives retinal input but projects to near-by midbrain, not to cortex (Sherman and Koch, 1998). It's a peculiarity of development in humans and other primates that the ventral LGN comes to lie *dorsal* to dorsal LGN. In its adult position, ventral LGN is sometimes called pregeniculate nucleus of thalamus (Jones, 1985a).

(If it helps the memory at all, ventral thalamus and epithalamus, both in the embryological sense, *don't* project to cortex, but *every* dorsal thalamic nucleus projects to cortex, albeit in different ways, depending on the dorsal thalamic nucleus we study. There are two corollary observations: 1. "virtually the whole cortex (allocortex as well as neocortex) receives a projection from the dorsal thalamus" and 2. "the nature of the projections . . . may vary from nucleus to nucleus and even among populations of cells in the same nucleus" [Jones, 1985b].)

*

Jones's dicta notwithstanding, note that LGN has no monosynaptic connection with cortex that we see *in this particular coronal section*. How do areas, to which LGN doesn't connect directly, influence what's to be done with visual information, for example, in exploring the environment?[4]

*

Frankly, it doesn't even look as if LGN is connected *to the rest of thalamus* in the image.

People talk about LGN's resemblance to Napoleon's hat (a simile that fails depending on your angle of view of Napoleon's head and the *bicorne* hat on it). Visually, doesn't it seem that the inverted "U" or vaguely sideways "S"-like shape of LGN in the image is physically at a distance from thalamus, displaced laterally? In fact, LGN *is* separated from the rest of thalamus by a medial ramus of the optic tract.

Both the optic tract and arteries supplying LGN enter at its hilus (the concavity of the inverted U); optic radiations leave from LGN's convexity–that is, from the dorsal aspect of LGN (Jones, 1985a).

*

LGN's proximity to the cerebral peduncle clues us to LGN's vascularization. As the posterior cerebral artery (PCA) courses posterolaterally around the peduncle, the branch-point of posterior communicating artery (PCOMM) is a landmark, assuming that we're not dealing with a PCA arising from the anterior circulation. In such a case

---

[4]   I have a passage from Sporns (2011) in mind: "Active exploration has physiological effects on neural responses. For example, whether a stimulus is presented passively or enters a neuron's receptive field as a result of a saccadic eye movement matters to the temporal response pattern of orientation-selective neurons in primate V1 [primary visual cortex]. Furthermore, human eye movements select locations in the visual environment that are relevant for particular perceptual or cognitive tasks. The selection of fixation points in a visual scene is determined by image content and the saliency of local visual features, as well as exploratory movements, and together these factors shape the statistics of visual inputs and direct the deployment of cognitive resources. *Outputs influence inputs*, and by directing fixation and visual gaze, motor neurons guiding eye, head, and body movements profoundly influence patterns of functional connectivity in the visual brain [my emphasis, p. 314]." "Output" in the passage refers mainly to movement presumably driven by frontal, not occipital, locations in brain.

of "fetal PCA," there's either an absent or very small contribution to PCA from the posterior circulation.

Proximal to the branch-point of PCOMM in most of us, there's a "P1" segment of PCA; a "P2" segment is distal to that branch point. Supply to LGN arises from posterior choroidal arteries of the distal P2 segment (viz., the posteromedial and posterolateral systems of Castaigne et al. [1981], who followed the lead of fellow Parisian Gerald Percheron; according to both Castaigne et al. and Percheron, there are a variable number of posterior choroidal arteries among people) (Bogousslavsky et al., 1988). There's been a thought that *anterior* choroidal artery, a branch of either internal carotid or middle cerebral in the anterior circulation, could supply part of LGN, but an older report using CT correlations found no LGN damage in a series of anterior choroidal artery infarcts (Schmahmann, 2003).

Yet, anterior choroidal artery supplies structures in the immediate vicinity of LGN, including hippocampus and the posterior limb of the internal capsule (among other structures). In addition, the posterolateral choroidal arteries off the P2 segment of PCA also supply hippocampus and medial temporal cortex (*inter alia*). Castaigne et al. (1981) have admitted that descriptions of thalamic vasculature are "somewhat sketchy," given significant inter-individual variability. They add, "one thalamic nucleus is usually not supplied by a single artery," and, in strokes involving the general area, "a lesion of a thalamic nucleus is most often only partial."

From a clinical point of view, an ischemic syndrome of LGN isn't reliable in terms of deficits that one observes. Homonymous field cuts aren't precise hemianopsias typically; there could be an associated contralateral sensory deficit, but not necessarily; there could be a memory deficit, or not (Schmahmann, 2003).

*

LGN receives bilateral retinal input, of course. It also receives homolateral, occipital cortical input: "Corticogeniculate axons in all species with a laminated nucleus [LGN] ramify densely in the interlaminar spaces between the cell laminae and appear to terminate primarily in parts of the laminae abutting on the spaces (Jones, 1985)." The interlaminar spaces are visible as thin strands of white in our coronal section.

If you rewind to the late 1960's, you can find a study by one of our seminar's imaginary participants regarding the *cortico*geniculate projection:

"A demonstration of the part that corticogeniculate fibers play in the organization of the visual system may depend to a large extent on defining the relationship that the cells of origin of the corticogeniculate fibers have to the origin of the many other corticofugal projections [*fugere*–to flee (in Latin), in this context, *from* cortex] arising in the visual cortex . . ." (Guillery, 1967).

That guess was prescient.

6

Categories of the First
and Higher Orders

F.A.H. mentioned ten thousand million separate cells (a lot of neurons) as opposed to a few million afferent fibres to them, but we can make things more meaningful to a person who wants to understand as much as she can without reference to overwhelming numbers or ratios.

As discussed in *The Visual Cortices*, the number of optic tract fibers heading to LGN is about the same as the number of neurons in an LGN (~one million). It turns out that there are vastly more inputs *from* primary visual cortex to LGN than there are LGN afferents *to* primary visual cortex. How can that be? And why is it so?

*

The thalamologists whom I'll cite often in this monograph tout a novel conception of their favorite subcortical structure:

> The dominant current view is that information initially arrives at cortex after being relayed through first order relays [such as LGN], and once in cortex it remains strictly at the cortical level, being analyzed and communicated among cortical areas strictly along hierarchical, possibly parallel (supposedly "where" and "what") corticocortical

pathways, until some instruction is ready to be sent to memory or to lower motor centers. . . .

> In contrast, our very different hypothesis, that corticocortical information transfer is relayed through . . . higher order thalamic nuclei, invests these relays with a critical function. Not only does it place the thalamus in a key role in corticocortical communication, but it also links that key role to the outputs that the relevant cortical areas are sending to the brainstem and spinal cord (Sherman and Guillery, 2006a).

Slipped into their discussion is a difference between "first" and "higher" orders of thalamic nuclei. This chapter addresses the two categories. Both have criteria for membership.

*

We can start with retinal data, which "relay" via LGN to cortex:

> . . . retinal input carries the main information for geniculocortical relay, and we have called this input *driver* input. What, then, is the role of the cortical input? . . . [I]t acts as a *modulator*, much like the classical cholinergic, noradrenergic, etc. modulators, affecting the gain and other aspects of retinogeniculate transmission. The main point here is that, whereas both the retinal and cortical inputs are glutamatergic, they have quite different functions and should not be grouped together (Sherman, 2017).

Using the visual pathway as a much studied touchstone, a retinal "driver," which is glutamatergic, inputs to LGN, *and* LGN receives other "modulator" input (also glutamatergic, but other neurotransmitters may be involved) from cortex and elsewhere. Most cortical input to LGN is modulatory. In terms of retinal input, drivers account for less than 10% of synapses in LGN (Sherman and Guillery, 2006, p. 11; Sherman, 2017).

Small in number, drivers drive large excitatory post-synaptic potentials at LGN synapses by activation of ionotropic glutamate receptors. On the other hand, modulation sets a stage for driving forces:

> Only 5–10% of the input to geniculate relay cells derives from the retina, which is the driving input. The rest is modulatory and derives from local inhibitory inputs, descending inputs from layer 6 of the visual cortex, and ascending inputs from the brainstem. These modulatory inputs control many features of retinogeniculate transmission. One such feature is the response mode, burst or tonic, of relay cells, which relates to the attentional demands at the moment. This response mode depends on membrane potential, which is controlled effectively by the modulator inputs. The lateral geniculate nucleus is a first-order relay, because it relays subcortical (i.e. retinal) information to the cortex for the first time. By contrast, the other main thalamic relay of visual information, the pulvinar region, is largely a higher-order relay, since much of it relays information from layer 5 of one cortical area to another. All thalamic relays receive a layer-6 modulatory input from cortex, but higher-order relays in addition receive a layer-5 driver input. Corticocortical processing may involve these corticothalamocortical 're-entry' routes to a far greater extent than previously appreciated (Sherman and Guillery, 2002).

There's a lot to unpack in the above passage. I'll focus on the cortical afferentation of thalamus, not the other way around.[5]

*

---

[5]   On the issue of how modulatory input influences the response mode of thalamus, suffice it to say that "burst" and "tonic" refer to physiological states of relay neurons that result not only from corticothalamic activity, but also intrinsic processing within thalamus—perhaps especially an interaction of nuclei, LGN representative among them, with (inhibitory) reticular nucleus of thalamus (Sherman and Guillery, 2006b).

We're used to teaching that LGN projects to layer IV of (mainly) primary visual cortex. Sherman and Guillery emphasize that *all thalamic nuclei*, whether of the first or higher order, *receive* layer VI projections.

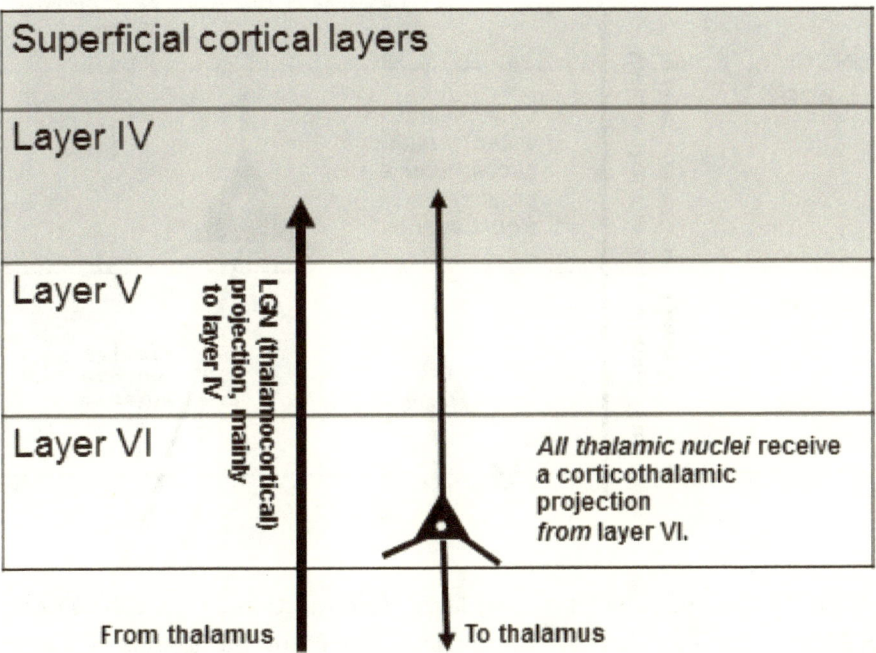

Note that layer VI neurons may project to layer IV (I've drawn a layer VI neuronal dendrite to illustrate the point simply, though it may be an axon that heads from layer VI to IV). The important thing to notice is that layer V, an output layer as layer VI is, plays no role, not yet. A distinction between first and higher order *thalamic* nuclei (e.g., LGN vs. pulvinar) has partly to do with afferentation *not* from layer VI.

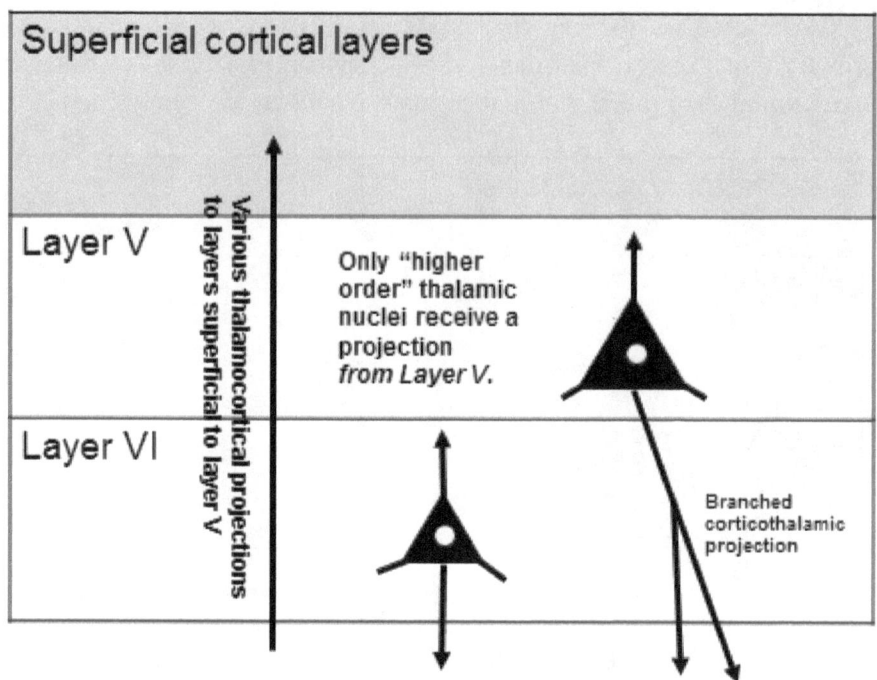

If all thalamic nuclei receive layer VI projections, then a first order nucleus is distinguished by: "subcortical" input[6] and the absence of a layer V projection to it.

Higher order thalamic nuclei may have first order features. Sherman (2017) talks about how superior colliculus dispatches driver input to pulvinar, for example. But higher order thalamic nuclei uniquely *receive* layer V input and they *project* to non-primary, "higher" cortical areas.

In other words, *a higher order thalamic nucleus is involved in cortex-to-cortex communication in a way that a first order nucleus isn't, because of different wirings.* LGN doesn't innervate primary auditory cortex and primary auditory cortex doesn't project to LGN. But other thalamic nuclei cross putative boundaries of function (e.g., the difference between sight and hearing). So, getting an idea what a higher order relay *does* requires that we appreciate: 1. the message that a thalamic nucleus receives and, vitally, *from where* and 2. the function of (a) cortical area(s) to which a higher order

---

[6]   "Subcortical" mainly means visual, auditory, or somatosensory input arising from retina, cochlea, or peripheral receptors in the body, but there are, of course, other subcortical (e.g., brainstem) projections to thalamus.

nucleus projects, to the degree that we can be confident about assigning a function to any area of cortex.

*

In this chapter, "categories" relate to neuroanatomical differences (e.g., the difference between LGN and pulvinar) that seem unassailable, based on work that's been done up until now. We don't refer to categories of experience based on our five senses, or the manner in which experience may be a function of very abstract categories such as quality, quantity, and relation.

In the back of my head, I wonder whether F.A.H. had an idea about categories like the latter three, but we'll get back to him later.

7

The Branched Projection

An observant reader notes that one aspect of the last diagram needs elaboration. In the lower right hand corner, there's a "branched corticothalamic projection," about which a book could be written (it has been written: Sherman and Guillery, 2013).

*

As in Part I, I'll go back in time. To 1950, specifically. We'll start there, but let's also anticipate where we'll conclude by this chapter's end; the second passage is from the book just mentioned:

> Axonal branching is a common feature of pathways in the central nervous system. An important property of such branching is that it serves to pass the *identical* message to all targets of the axon. That is, the same pattern of action potentials passes down all branches to their terminals. This does not mean that all targets respond identically, because different synaptic properties likely exist at different terminals. Nonetheless, axonal branching is the most effective way to share a common message from one neuron to multiple targets (Sherman, 2017).

*

The focus for us has been on the thalamic inputs, the motor outputs, and the transthalamic outputs to cortex. This is quite different from the question more generally addressed, which concerns the cognitive, perceptual, or behavioral circumstances during which a particular cortical area can be shown to be active on the basis of increased blood flow or other signs of increased activity. We have described this approach as evidence-based phrenology, because, unlike the old phrenology, it is based on the action of the brain itself and so it clearly relates to what the brain is doing and serves to localize certain definable functions. However, the functions identified for any one cortical area by these means are often not linked to any defined inputs from the world or the body nor are they linked to any defined outputs from that cortical area (Sherman and Guillery, 2013a).

*

Back to 1950.

*

Their wording is tortured in translation, but the German authors of a dense paper published that year address a subject that should obsess any thalamologist. Regarding the relationship between input and output, they write: "We do not enquire into the relations between a given afference (input) and the efference (output) to which it gives rise . . . but rather start with the efference and ask: what happens after the efference has caused changes in the organism via the effectors, and then is reverberated back into the CNS by way of the receptors, as afference? This type of afference which is caused by the efference itself we shall call rea[f]ference (Von Holst and Mittelstaedt, 1950)." I'll invite the reader to stick with terms as defined, though it's probably already clear that I pulled an early paper on the concept of an *efference copy.*

To summarize:

1. 1. *Afference equals Input* (e.g., peripheral input to ventral posterior nucleus of thalamus related to somatosensation).
2. 2. *Efference equals Output* (e.g., primary motor cortex output to the periphery).
3. 3. *Which comes first, the afference or the efference?* (The authors don't refer to something like a normal monosynaptic reflex, in which obvious input–a strike with a hammer at a tendon–yields immediate, stereotyped output.) Rather, they ask: *What if you can't tell which came first?*[7]
4. 4. You could take a point in time at which some effector (e.g., a muscle), acting in response to input, has caused a change of the body in relation to the environment, and that change is communicated–inputted to CNS. That's *reafference*, as described in the passage.

Now the authors elaborate: consider some CNS center, they suggest, which "services" an effector. This center, or hierarchy of centers, produces an output or efference. In addition to *that* efference, however, it also "causes a *strictly correlated neuronal process* (e.g., by a change of activity which spreads, after a certain temporal delay, into neighboring ganglia) called the *efference copy*" (my emphases, Von Holst and Mittelstaedt, 1950).

How does all the above look from the perspective of either cortex or thalamus?

*

Guillery (in many publications, but I'll concentrate on Guillery, 2005) sets himself to answer the last question.

A few pages into the 2005 paper, he asks us to think about the very early brain, as in this image, in which myelin is dark; the specimen is from a one-day old infant studied by Paul Emil Flechsig in late 19th century Leipzig:

---

7   The authors acknowledge that a change in afference (input) may not be a direct consequence of efference (output), "but rather results from external stimulation." They term such a situation as an "exafference."

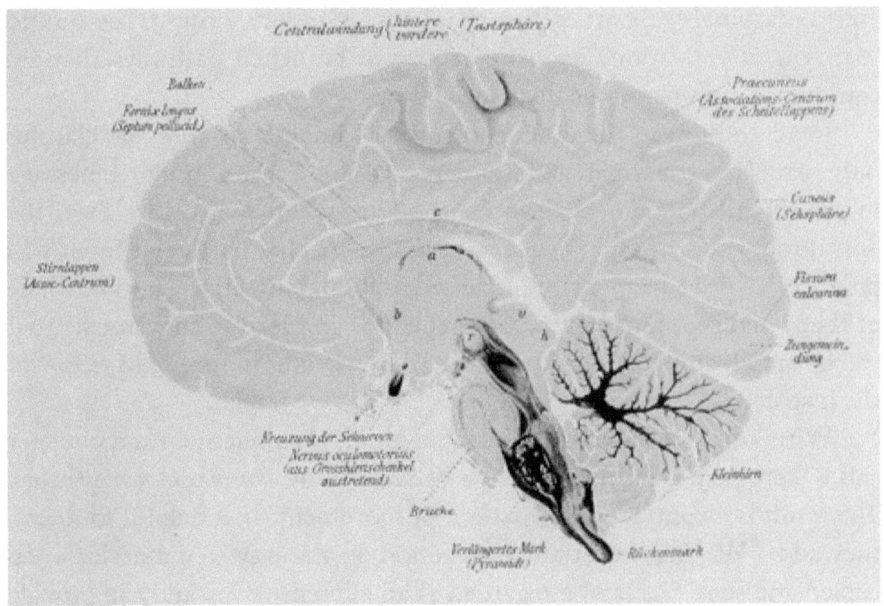

Aside from some subcortical myelin, a shadow across corpus callosum (c), a bit more darkness in what looks like stria medullaris of thalamus (*a*) and perhaps mammillothalamic tract (*b*), and the dark optic chiasm and third cranial nerve in the ventral midline, the appearance of this one-day-old brain is that of an unmyelinated prosencephalon and a much more myelinated rhombencephalon, with the exception of the pons ("*Brücke*").

Sensory afferents may reach thalamus, but thalamocortical pathways can only be considered immature on day one of life and well into the first year. The same immaturity pertains to descending tracts.

An infant learns "the significance of a particular dorsal root input, [but] the messages must be understood to represent not just the tactile or proprioceptive changes represented by the discharge of the peripheral receptors, but also a particular pattern of activation of complex spinal and supraspinal [subcortical] mechanisms," Guillery writes.[8] The link to "patterns of activation" happens by way of branched pathways that are common if not ubiquitous in all animals.

Read and reread the 2005 paper, yet its underlying message clarifies only years later (Sherman and Guillery, 2013b): "If we consider a message to the spinal motor mechanisms, no matter whether it comes from the dorsal root or from higher centers in the brain, that particular input will produce not just a particular muscle contraction, but will engage the whole of the spinal or brainstem pattern generator and lead to movements that can be anticipated to a significant extent by a center in receipt of a copy of the instructions."

With Von Holst and Mittelstaedt in mind, what Sherman and Guillery call a "corollary" sensory discharge behaves *in the manner of a reafference.* The result is a contraction or pattern of movement. In a helpful footnote, they add: "We stress that any instruction on the way to a muscle, when copied and sent . . ., can be regarded as an efference copy and can provide early information about forthcoming movements. The nonmotor ascending branches of dorsal root inputs can serve this function and invariably provide information ahead of the information produced when the muscle contraction moves the receptor (Sherman and Guillery, 2013a)."

If we now add mature and myelinated prosencephalon to the discussion, does an interaction between afference, efference, reafference, and efference copy much change?

*

----

[8]   There's a way in which, even in 2005, Guillery subverts the separation we teach between sensory and motor systems. In 2013, Sherman and Guillery discuss *tabes dorsalis* as an affliction of dorsal root axons to spinal cord, with emphasis on how those axons *branch*: "One branch, ascending in the posterior columns, carries messages to the thalamus and cortex, providing the information that is needed for perceptions about tactile inputs and about the position and movements of the limbs. . . . The other branch, the one that innervates the spinal pattern generators is not, strictly speaking, "sensory" at all from the point of view of the patient or the clinician. It provides the same afferent information to the central pattern generators of the spinal cord, serving both as a feedback in the control of movements and also providing information about changes in the environment (Sherman and Guillery, 2013b)."

Guillery's 2005 paper has the title "Anatomical Pathways that Link Perception and Action," but it could have been called "Input, Output, and Thalamocortex." He relies on his driver vs. modulator distinction, of course:

> A driver input to the thalamus is the one that carries the actual message that is transmitted to the cortex, and it differs significantly from a modulatory input, which can modify the way in which the message is transmitted, or can change the nature of the message in particular, often subtle ways. Although the drivers represent considerably less than 10% of synapses in their thalamic relays, where they have been tested, silencing them produces a loss of the receptive field properties that characterize their thalamic relays.

Reference to receptive field properties places us squarely in the domain of sensory input,[9] which must connect, structurally, to output, according to Guillery.

The respective anatomies of layer V and VI projections to thalamus speak to that connection, as Sherman and Guillery re-emphasize years later:

> Many layer 5 cells have axons that do not go to the thalamus but go to other centers. The important point to stress here is that the layer 5 cells that do project to the thalamus all appear to have long descending branches that innervate one or another of the lower motor centers (striatum, superior colliculus, pontine nuclei, pontine reticular formation, or spinal cord . . .). The contrast with layer 6 corticothalamic axons is important. The axons from layer 6 cells form a large part of the input to all thalamic nuclei. They send a modulatory signal as a

---

[9]   The receptive field properties of thalamic nuclear cells may or may not differ from those of cortical cells. Layer VI neurons feedback to thalamic nuclei, but the cortical cells' receptive field properties aren't those of the thalamic nuclei. If, for example, layer VI cortical input to LGN were interrupted, retinal driver input from LGN to primary visual cortex wouldn't be eliminated.

feedback message to the thalamus. They send branches
to the thalamic reticular nucleus but send no branches
beyond the diencephalon. . . . [L]ayer 5 cells do not have
branches that innervate the thalamic reticular nucleus and
have long descending branches to brainstem motor centers
(Sherman and Guillery, 2013b).

Earlier in this chapter, we heard a jibe about the "evidence-based
phrenology" of functional imaging. "Functional connectivity" just
isn't structure, neither for Guillery nor even among those who study
thalamocortex functionally (e.g., Zhang et al., 2010).

Structurally, layer V projections pass to either to thalamus or output
centers in brainstem or elsewhere. The point of this chapter, however, is
that the projection *branches*, thereby passing an identical message to all
axonal termini. A repeated datum, in the sensory domain, constitutes a
corollary discharge and, in the motor domain, an efference copy.

Either way, a faithful identity of transmission is the virtue of a branched
projection.

8

A Loaded Comment

I notice, J.VN. said, that we tend *not* to process external visual, auditory, and other sensory data while asleep, whereas when awake, there is no such non-tendency.

People couldn't decide whether he was serious or not.

I sleep with my eyes closed, P.G.-R. said.

And on waking, J.VN. continued (as if talking to himself), a gate opens. Then we have . . . first order, higher order, etc., as we've heard, rather like a long calculation or series of individual calculations. And:

> . . . in the course of long calculations, not only do errors add up but also those committed early in the calculation are amplified by the latter parts of it; therefore, considerably higher precision is needed than the physical nature of the problem would by itself appear to require (Von Neumann, 2000).

After scribbling numbers on the whiteboard in our room, he concluded that a ten- or twelve-decimal precision wouldn't exaggerate the requirements of an "automaton" as reliable as the brain is, especially in a state of wakeful awareness. "This conclusion was well worth working out just because of, rather than in spite of, its absolute implausibility," he said (Von Neumann, 2000).

If such arithmetical "depth" (J.VN.'s word) can't plausibly be achieved by a brain, there must be some other, perhaps logical or *structural* depth to it.

I can address that, P.G.-R. said.

PART III

9

Her Psychic Cells

Published in 2002, Goldman-Rakic's homage to Cajal, "The 'Psychic Cell' of Ramón y Cajal," proves not to be an historical study so much as an explanation of her and her lab's interest in the prefrontal cortex, particularly of the rhesus monkey (*Macaca mulatta*).

She refers to cortex anterior to the superior arcuate sulcus in the rhesus brain, along on the dorsal and ventral banks of the principal sulcus. It's frontal lobe (yes), but, in particular, the part of it very much anterior/rostral to central sulcus:

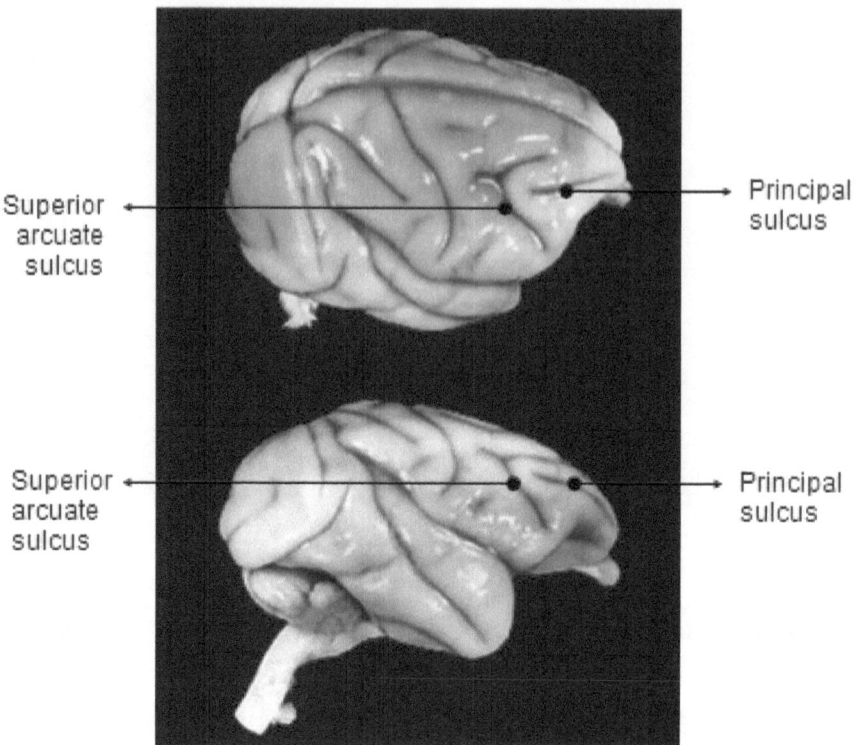

Superior arcuate sulcus → Principal sulcus

Superior arcuate sulcus → Principal sulcus

The oblique view in the upper image alerts us to the fact (in *M. mulatta*) that cortex dorsal to the principal sulcus extends towards the interhemispheric fissure thence onto the medial surface of a hemibrain. So, we also refer to cortex dorsal and even a bit posterior to the superior arcuate sulcus (*and* we refer to prefrontal cortex ventral to principal sulcus extending to the inferior surface of the hemibrain). I omit medial and inferior views of this brain for simplicity, but the point is that Goldman-Rakic's attention riveted on the cortical pole opposite from occiput.

*

Cajal referred to pyramidal neurons anywhere in the cortex as "psychic cells" endowed with uncanny capacity. Goldman-Rakic's specific interest in *prefrontal* pyramidal neurons had been influenced by primate research done largely by John Fulton and Carlyle Jacobsen, both of whom worked at Yale decades before Goldman-Rakic did. (Fulton and Jacobsen, incidentally, spurred Egas Moniz to attempt frontal lobotomies in humans for the treatment of psychiatric conditions. Moniz, from Lisbon, attended a London conference where he learned about their results in 1935.[10])

In 1936, Jacobsen published that lesions of frontal association areas resulted in a specific learning problem having to do with context. If all cues were present in the immediate environment to accomplish a task, monkeys–either with or without surgically produced prefrontal lesions–had no difficulty with successful completion. But under conditions "in which certain essential cues had to be recalled from recent experience (delayed response)," post-surgical monkeys couldn't complete successfully at all–indeed, "[t]he subjects failed in this test with delays as short as one or two seconds," Jacobsen wrote (1936). The delayed response task, Goldman-Rakic explains, "require[s] animals to hold an item of information in mind for several seconds and to update a mental representation of that input on a moment by moment basis (Goldman-Rakic, 2003)."

Jacobsen compared his primate data with results in the rat. He speculated that there might be "a different plan of organization in the primate brain, an organization in which specialized association areas mediate the more complex integrative functions which are subserved in the rat by the cortex *as a whole* (my emphasis; Jacobsen, 1936)."

In the last chapter, J.VN. wondered about some non-serial, non-arithmetical logic–a "depth," as he put it–unique to brains. Jacobsen might've piqued J.VN.'s curiosity had the two ever communicated. For the primate brain, its "depth" might *localize* to prefrontal cortex and to neurons there.

*

---

[10]   Moniz was inspired by the case of "Becky" (Tierney, 2000): "Prior to surgery, one of the animals, Becky, reacted in a highly emotional way to the tests, at times refusing to enter the chamber or becoming enraged when she made an error and was denied the food reward. However, following bilateral removal of the frontal lobes, she became strikingly more cooperative, approaching the task willingly and displaying no frustration despite making far more errors than she had prior to surgery. Jacobson and Fulton . . . focused on the learning deficits that followed frontal lobe removal, but it was the mention of emotional changes that captured Moniz's attention. Fulton . . . later wrote that Moniz arose after the presentation and questioned, 'if frontal lobe removal prevents the development of experimental neuroses in animals and eliminates frustrational [*sic*] behavior, why would it not be feasible to relieve anxiety states in man by surgical means?'"

Goldman-Rakic wondered about how information is represented in prefrontal neurons. In a related way, our curiosity has to do with how information gets to areas with the depth, capacity, or specialization for particular cognitive tasks. Also: how *does* information pass from the very back to the very front in a brain? Her lab addressed the issue, and we turn to that work in chapter twelve, after we discuss basic thalamic nuclear anatomy in chapters ten and eleven.

Before we leave our re-introduction to P.G.-R., one wonders why Cajal used the word "psychic," with all its connotations of extrasensory perception, when he fundamentally referred just to the pyramidal cells he visualized in his preparations. He could have just called them "large."

The simple answer is that he understood something distinctive about them, certainly in comparison to non-pyramidal cells of cortex. Goldman-Rakic says the difference between those cells relates not only to distinct neuronal morphologies (e.g., long vs. local axons) or types of respective neurotransmission (glutamatergic vs. GABAergic), but also to a prefrontal pyramidal cell's "extensive sensory monosynaptic connections with the higher order sensory cortices" and its "inferred ability to hold information transiently 'on-line' (Goldman-Rakic, 2003)."

Her own definition of "psychic" is revisionist; for her, the word has to do with a "higher order" and memory.

10

A Serviceable Atlas of Thalamic Nuclei

Part A

If you plan a career in human stereotactic neurosurgery, it might be worth the investment to obtain Schaltenbrand and Wahren's *Atlas for Stereotaxy of the Human Brain*, in which you can find extraordinary detail about thalamus in images that measure up to 12 by 16 inches. For the careerist studying *M. mulatta* as Goldman-Rakic did, maybe a copy of Jerzy Olszewski's *The Thalamus of Macaca Mulatta* should be on your shelf.

Reading either, you quickly encounter a problem with nomenclatures: in humans, there's Schaltenbrand and Wahren's, Hassler's, Van Buren and Borke's, Cecile and Oskar Vogt's, and Walker's, all of which differ from Olszewski's, which was specific for the monkey. Further: all the above naming systems differ in minor and major ways from the one most familiar to American students–which is essentially Walker's or perhaps Jones's (Jones tried to use the same names for thalamic nuclei across many animal species; Walker studied primates).

Can we try something simpler?

*

We'll identify structures of thalamus that we can actually see without a microscope. Schaltenbrand and Wahren say it's often the case, especially in unstained preparations, that even large nuclei have to be lumped together

41

(Schaltenbrand and Wahren, 1977a). Nuclei sheathed in white matter tend to stand out; we'll study images in which white matter stains darkly.

We'll stick with coronal slices, so that for any given section we have a sense of what happens when passing from the dorsal to ventral surface of a thalamus. Specific image sources, all available on-line for public use, are provided in "References." On behalf of the seminar, I acknowledge with thanks the treasure that is "The Human Brain Atlas," part of the brain collections of the National Museum of Health and Medicine, Michigan State University, and the University of Wisconsin.

Our nomenclature is Jones's (Jones, 1985, see pp. 83-84 specifically), but we also try to abide by names used in studies of rat thalamus (see "Thalamocortex" in my *Beneath the Cortical Surface*).

*

We move from front to back.

First cut's location: level of the amygdalae, posterior to anterior commissure.

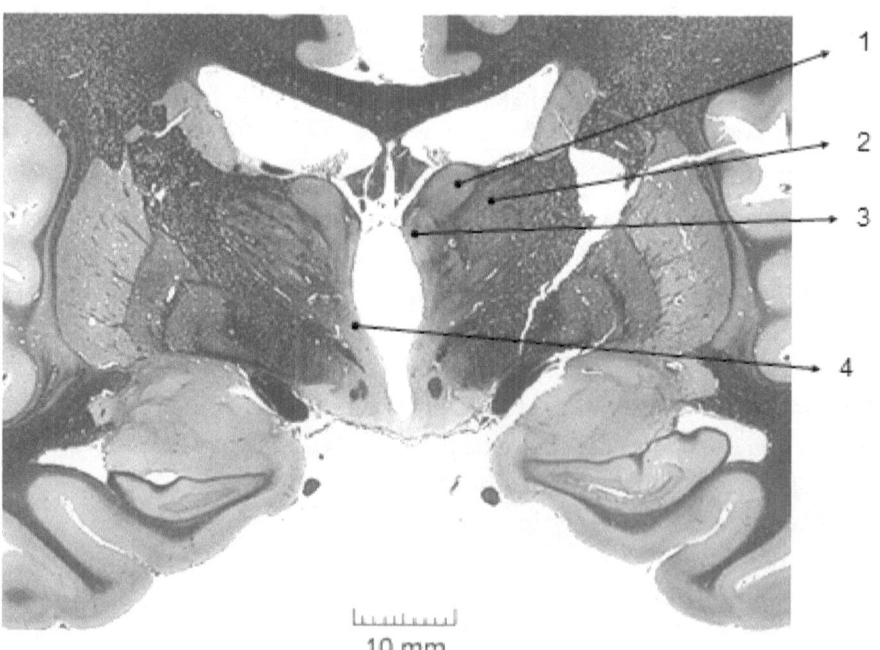

10 mm

The procedure of this chapter isn't to name structures to memorize them. Instead, I suggest thinking through–*describing*–the anatomy.

At the rostral pole of thalamus–where we are in the image–there's physical proximity between *anterior nuclei* (there are several of them, marked together as "1") and *ventral anterior nucleus* (Hassler's nucleus latero*polaris*, marked as "2," as opposed to his nucleus *ventrooralis* [ventral lateral nucleus]).

Lateral to "2," one might expect to see a bit of *reticular nucleus*, which forms a lateral shell along much of thalamus–from tip to rear of thalamus. Reticular nucleus always lies just medial to the internal capsule, but I can't readily see it in the image. So, I don't label it.

"1" (look carefully at its lateral edge) and "2" are separated by a white matter tract which passes ventrally, the *mammillothalamic tract*. While true that anterior nuclear group is bounded by fibers of the *internal medullary lamina* of thalamus, in this anterior coronal section, a fiber tract passing inferiorly from "1" can only be mammillothalamic tract.

Deep and medial to "1," it appears that there's uninterrupted grey matter which frames third ventricle and which extends towards hypothalamus. There are two parts of that medial grey that look different from each other: "3" is *parataenial nucleus* (*taenium* refers to a ribbon; there's a relationship between the nucleus and the *taenia tecta* of rat forebrain) and "4" is *paraventricular nucleus* of thalamus (not of hypothalamus).

Parataenial nucleus merges posteriorly with medial dorsal nucleus (Jones, 1985, p. 664), the latter not yet visible, because we are too anterior in this section. Paraventricular nucleus, which Jones includes among *epithalamic* nuclei (Jones, 1985, pp. 737ff.), eventually merges with periaqueductal grey of the midbrain.

Just because grey matter is located medially, it's not the case that it therefore belongs to the group called "medial nuclei" of thalamus (anterior nucleus looks rather medial in this section, but it's *more anterior* than medial)–and a name like "ventral anterior" doesn't perforce mean that the nucleus can only be found ventrally. In discussing "medial nuclei," the most obvious and perhaps most important of them is medial dorsal nucleus, which has enlarged over evolution and is especially large in primates and humans (see next image).

The phylogeny of anterior nuclear group, which is also associated with memory-related circuitry, is complex, with certain anterior nuclei enlarging and others disappearing across species (Jones, 1985, pp. 675ff.).

"1" is physically close to *lateral dorsal nucleus*, though I'm not convinced that I can identify a discrete grey matter collection lateral and dorsal to "1" and "2." Because anterior and lateral dorsal nuclei share many of the same limbic connections in various species, the argument has been made that lateral dorsal nucleus should be considered part of the anterior group (Jones, 1985, p. 675).

*

Second cut's location: level of midbrain; red nuclei *aren't* obvious in this cut.

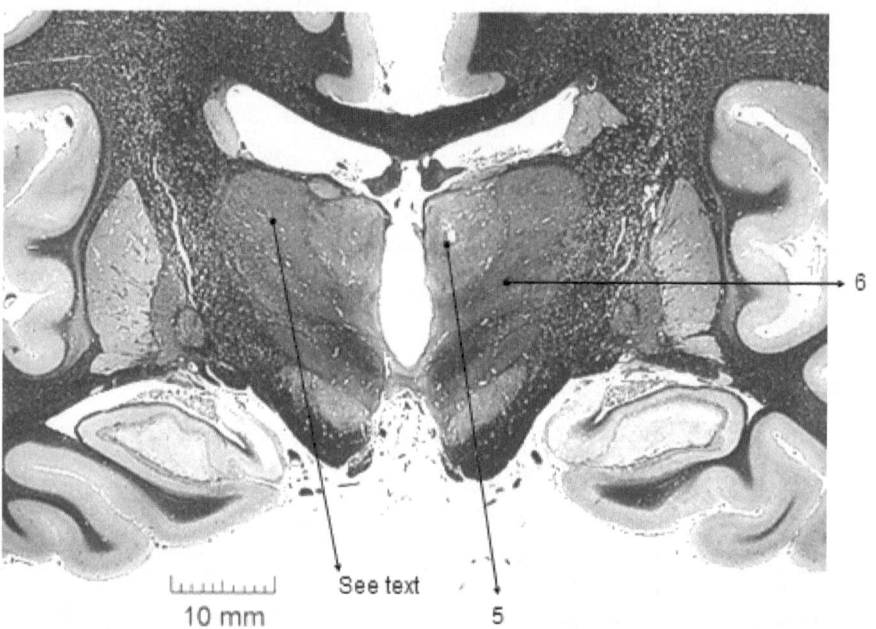

10 mm   See text   5   6

Two new structures are marked "5" and "6."

The appearance of medial thalamus has changed. Deep to the anterior nuclear group, there are wisps of black that form a curved line separating medial from lateral thalamic nuclei.

"5" is *medial dorsal nucleus*, bounded laterally by the internal medullary lamina. Medial dorsal

nucleus is "usually large and occupies up to two-thirds of the length of thalamus" (Jones, 1985, p. 649).

Jones describes its connection with frontal lobe based on work dating to the late 19th century (1985, p. 658): "[V]on Monakow (1895) in the cat and Minkowski (1924) in the monkey . . . pointed out, from retrograde degeneration studies, the association between mediodorsal [medial dorsal] nucleus and the frontal lobe. This was confirmed by Le Gros Clark and Boggon [~1930's]. . . in the rat and by Walker [1940's] who, using the retrograde degeneration method, related the nucleus to frontal granular cortex." Frontal *granular* cortex differs from *agranular* cortex; the latter characterizes motor and pre-motor domains of frontal lobe.

A whole thalamus on either side can be divided essentially in two: medially, there's the massive medial dorsal nucleus; *lateral* to internal medullary lamina, I'm tempted to indicate a visible difference between the dorsolateral and ventrolateral aspects of the big lateral thalamic half. You can find atlases (e.g., Schaltenbrand and Wahren, 1977, plate 27) specifying a *lateral posterior nucleus* situated above *ventral lateral nucleus*, the latter marked as "6" (we have moved posteriorly, so ventral anterior nucleus has passed from view). Yet Jones, on whom I obviously rely, teaches me that there's a kind of *intercalation* of ventral anterior, ventral lateral, ventral posterior, lateral dorsal, and lateral posterior nuclei:

> In monkeys, apes, and man, the lateral posterior nucleus is relatively small . . . .. The nucleus lies on the dorsal surface of the ventral posterior nucleus against the external medullary lamina [which separates lateral thalamic nuclei from reticular nucleus], overlain by the backwards-curving tails of the posterior ventral lateral and lateral dorsal nuclei (1985, p. 531).

With reference to where ventral anterior nucleus ends and ventral lateral nucleus begins, there's also a fuzzy boundary (in the absence of magnified sections stained for neurons), but one begins to understand why ventral anterior and ventral lateral nuclei are often considered as a single, ventral-motoric complex, given that both project to agranular frontal cortex.

Jones's narration helps me more than atlas pictures:

> The ventral lateral occupies much of the ventral nuclear mass anterior to the ventral posterior nucleus. In

small mammals such as rodents and even in the cat, it extends almost to the anterior pole of the ventral nuclear mass, separated only by a small ventral anterior nucleus. In the majority of mammals it extends for some distance posteriorly along the medial and/or dorsal surface of the ventral posterior nucleus, usually reaching the lateral posterior nucleus. . . . In primates parts of its dorsal surface reach to the dorsal surface of the thalamus (1985, p. 378).

*

Seminar organizer's prerogative: I offer a chapter break here.

11

Serviceable Atlas, Part B

Third cut's location: midbrain again, now with some pons in the section; red nuclei are obvious in this cut.

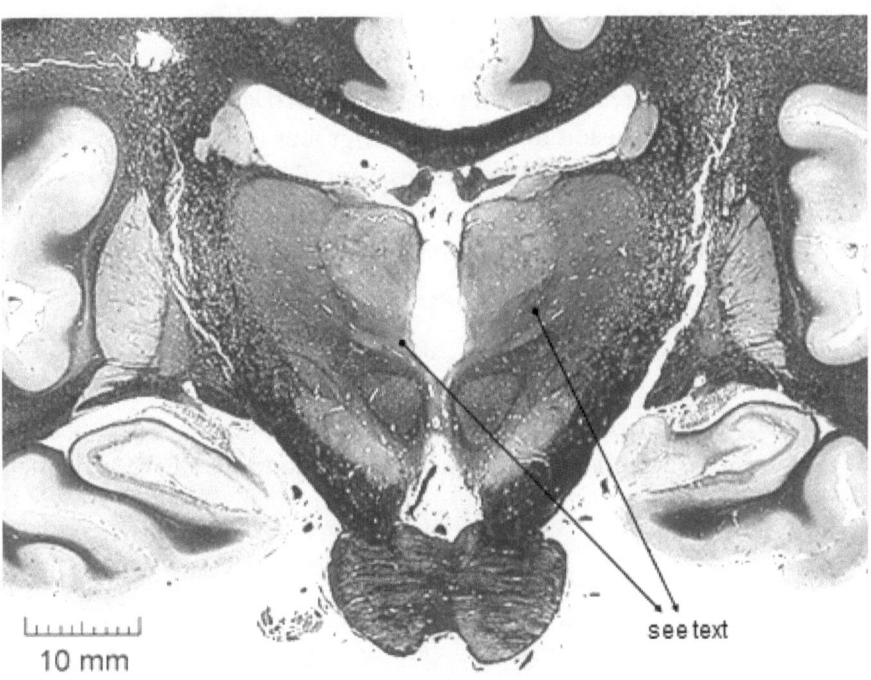

10 mm

see text

Tracing the lateral edge of either medial dorsal nucleus ventrally (i.e., along fibers of the internal medullary lamina), it appears a darkness widens on approach to the midline. There's discrete grey matter below medial dorsal nuclei.

Gazing to either side of the third ventricle dorsal to the red nuclei, one *might* appreciate why early anatomists described two wings of central grey matter that spread from the midline. I say "might," because maybe you don't see any such thing, but I draw attention to the area, because of work that relates very midline nuclei as well as the intralaminar nuclei to arousal and awareness (e.g., Van der Werf et al., 2002). Intralaminar nuclei are bounded entirely by the internal medullary lamina—we'll look at a prominent intralaminar nucleus in the next image.

For now, however, we simply acknowledge a cluster of medial nuclei that are deep/ventral to medial dorsal nucleus and medial to both ventral lateral and ventral posterior nuclei (the last two both lateral to the internal medullary lamina): "The *ventral medial complex* is a group of nuclei, some of which have ill-defined borders, mainly extending along the medial borders of the ventral lateral complex and ventral posterior nucleus and across the midline beneath the internal medullary lamina. . . . [I]ts several component nuclei are probably best identified in nonprimates, though part of the reason for their apparent omission from standard atlases of primate thalami stems from their inclusion in other nuclear groups (Jones, 1985, p. 411)."

Among other functional associations, ventral medial complex has been implicated in taste sensation, and just lateral to that complex, in microscopic sections, one typically finds cells comprising the *ventral posterior medial nucleus* (related to sensation from the face).

*

Fourth cut's location: level of posterior commissure, decussating fibers of the superior cerebellar peduncles in high midbrain, and the geniculate nuclei of thalamus.

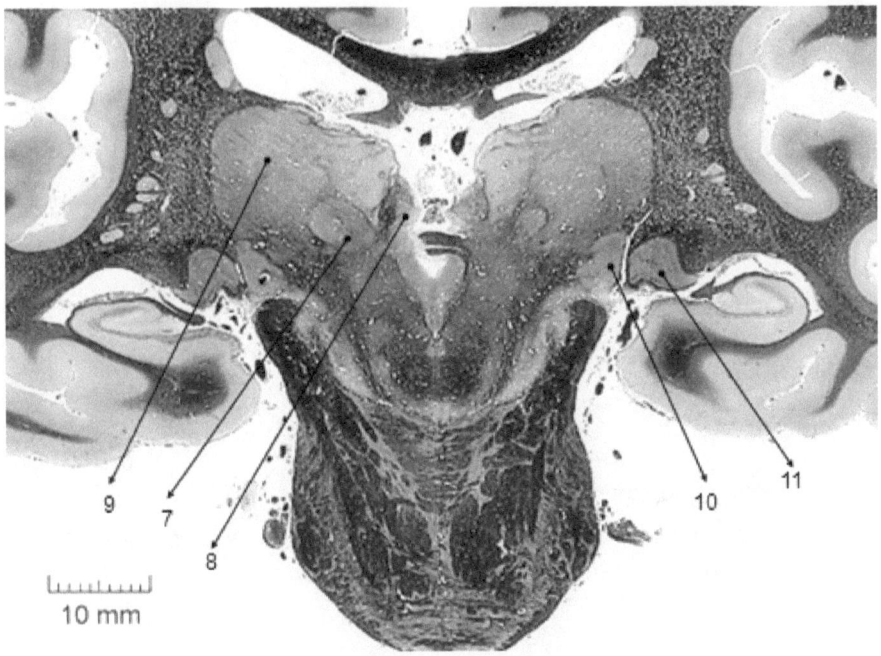

10 mm

Medial dorsal nucleus is still visible, even though we're posterior in thalamus.

*

Jules Bernard Luys first used the term *centre médian* to describe the structure marked as "**7**" (for clarity, I boldface our numbers in discussing this image, but will italicize Luys').[11]

It's worth a moment, so as to gain a better sense of our "**7**," to understand what Luys thought of the structure he marks as "*9*" in his 1882 textbook: a "sensory middle center (*centre médian sensitif*)." His textbook enjoyed multiple editions and is available in English translation; here is figure 5 in

---

[11] Jones (1985, p. 621) is usefully pedantic about the name *centre médian*, which ". . . is, of course, Luys's term, introduced in 1865 as the result of Luys's researches on the human brain. *Nucleus centrum medianum* is neither good Latin nor correct in the sense in which Luys envisaged this 'center' operating." Luys described centers, not nuclei, though he sometimes likens his centers to ganglia. Jones mainly wants to avoid confusion between *centre médian* and what has been Anglicized as "centromedian" nucleus. The latter is easily confused with midline nuclei located ventral to the medial dorsal nucleus.

the fifth French edition (Luys, 1882, p. 25 in the fifth French edition, p. 31 in the English translation):

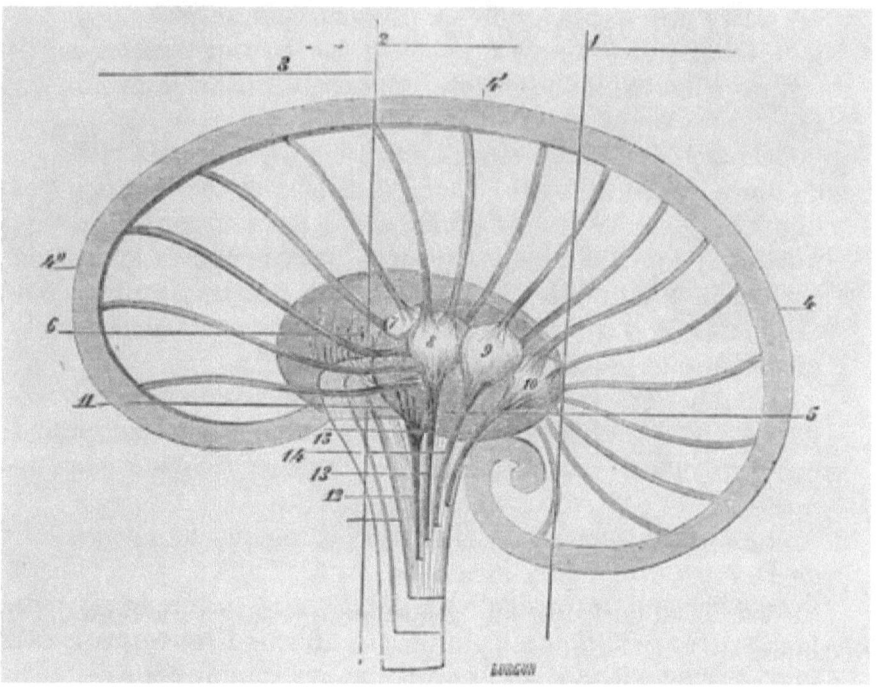

Luys' schematization describes deep centers *7-10*. The centers' specific names are: an anterior olfactory center (*7*), a middle optical center (*8*), a middle (somato)sensory center (*9*), and a posterior acoustic center (*10*).

Luys' is an early, perhaps the first (Krieg, 1953), characterization of thalamus as a sensory hub related not only to cortex, as the stylized thalamocortical projections illustrate in the image, but also to *corpus striatum*, which is depicted as the larger of two central grey ovals in the image. Luys refers to *corpus striatum* and thalamus as "natural poles around which all the nervous elements gravitate" (1882, p. 46 in the English translation).

There seems nevertheless to be something unique to thalamus, related to its "node-edge" or "hub-spoke" arrangement. Luys indicates four thalamic nodes and a fan-like thalamocortical emanation.

*

Based on contemporary, comparative study among vertebrates, *centre médian* derives from a discrete intralaminar nucleus found close to it, the *parafascicular nucleus*. In primates and humans, compared to rabbits, marsupials, bats, rats, shrews, and hoofed animals, *centre médian* is disproportionately large (Jones, 1985, pp. 615-625). Recent study has found that *centre médian*-parafascicular (CM/Pf) complex provides "massive, functionally organized glutamatergic inputs to the whole striatal complex [a thalamo*striatal* projection]," and, in terms of clinical relevance, significant loss of neurons in the CM/Pf complex has been observed in progressive supranuclear palsy, Huntington's disease, and Parkinson's disease (Smith et al., 2009).

*

Medial to "**7**" is a patch of black (*fasciculus retroflexus* or the *habenula-interpeduncular tract*) that contains output from habenula ("**8**"). As discussed in chapter 9 of *Beneath the Cortical Surface*, habenula inhibits midbrain dopamine centers under adverse conditions–e.g., an unforeseen danger in one's vicinity.

*

What does "**9**" indicate? It's a sincere question. It could be part of *ventral posterior lateral nucleus* or perhaps pulvinar or part of the so-called *posterior complex*, which "has usually been regarded as the anterior portion of the *medial geniculate nucleus* [the latter marked as "**10**" in our coronal section] or as part of the ventral posterior nucleus" (Jones, 1985, p. 585).

In the lateral half of thalamus in this section, I see subtle black streaks that aren't artifactual: they could be ascending lemniscal fibers; yet pulvinar, as we'll see in the next image, also has linear arrays of fibers, especially laterally.

One could perform single-unit studies to determine an answer, as was done in seminal work from Baltimore, circa 1960:

> In recording from single units throughout a large part of the posterior complex of barbiturate-anesthetized cats, [Gian] Poggio and [Vernon] Mountcastle remarked on the great difference between their receptive field properties and those of the adjoining ventral posterior nucleus. The

majority of ventral posterior neurons . . . possess small, contralateral receptive fields and respond to only one type of peripheral stimulus. That is, they are place and modality specific. By contrast, 60% of the units recorded in the posterior complex . . . responded not to gentle mechanical stimulation of the body but to cuts, pinpricks, and other stimuli that threatened destruction of tissue. *Many of the remaining neurons could be activated by gentle mechanical stimulation of skin or hairs but all neurons had extremely large receptive fields covering much of the contralateral, ipsilateral, and even both sides of the body* (my emphasis indicates my astonishment over bilateral, large receptive fields; Jones, 1985, p. 598).

I can't say definitively what our "**9**" is, but I've mentioned the reasonable options.

While *medial* ("**10**") and *lateral geniculate* ("**11**") *nuclei* seem obvious enough to the eye, the labeling doesn't speak to "**11**" as a first-order thalamic relay in Sherman and Guillery's sense, whereas the medial geniculate complex (comprised of several nuclei distinguishable microscopically) is higher order.[12]

*

Our last section includes superior colliculus.

I indicate *pulvinar* with a white "P" to the left side, but it's worth noting that pulvinar in primates and humans is very much larger than the homologous structure in rodents. So, we visualize only a part of it on either side in the image.

---

[12]   I suggest in chapter 12 of *Beneath the Cortical Surface* that there are only three first-order thalamic nuclei: lateral geniculate, ventral posterior lateral, and ventral posterior medial. If so, then the majority of thalamic nuclei are higher order, period. (Medial geniculate nucleus turns out to be a complex, higher-order entity, based on the argument of that chapter.)

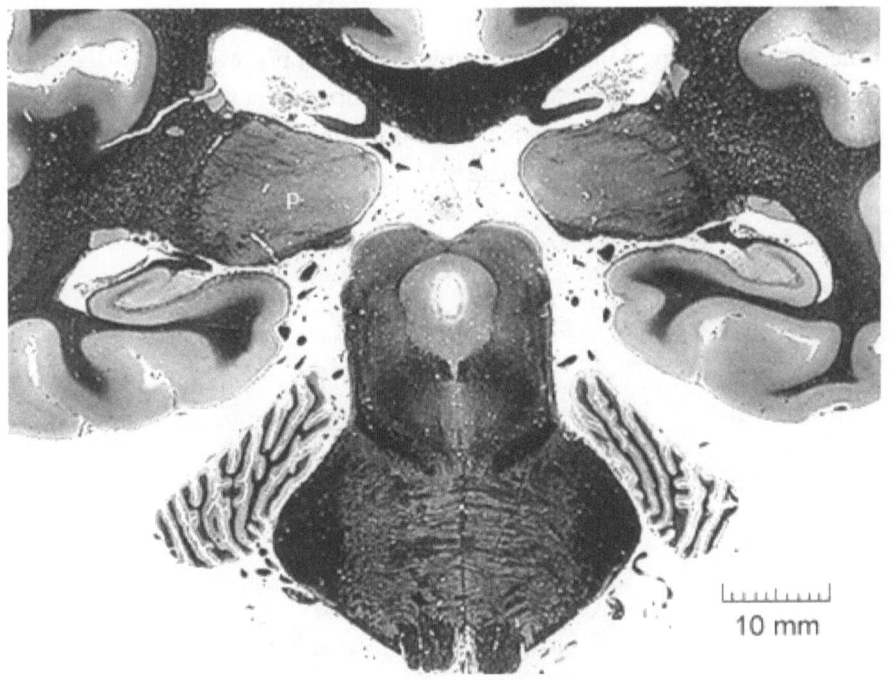

10 mm

An increased cortical surface area dedicated to vision, from extrastriate occipital lobe to parietal and much of temporal lobes, is a major development in mammalian evolution (Van Essen, 1979). Accompanying that enlargement, pulvinar in humans and primates accounts for up to a third of total thalamic volume (Lakatos et al., 2016).

Traditionally, pulvinar has been associated with a *tectothalamic pathway* that bypasses lateral geniculate nucleus (retina to superior colliculus/ pretectum to lateral posterior nucleus-pulvinar complex, to extrastriate visual cortex).

Look at the lateral half of pulvinar: neurons in lateral pulvinar are "broken up into linear arrays by the bundles of fibers of the so-called *corticotectal tract* that traverse the nucleus" (Jones, 1985, p. 537).

Cortex projects to tectum (a reminder that there's "top-down" processing in brains); tectum links to pulvinar; pulvinar projects to large areas of cortex).

*

In what way do prefrontal cortical locales, discussed in our chapter nine, come into play? One asks not only in terms of posterior-most thalamus (pulvinar prominent in it) and its relationship with anterior-most cortex, but also with regard to thalamocortical function involving *any* of the nuclei described in this and the last chapter.

12

Memory Field

Let's say that one identifies then records from a single neuron of layer V in prefrontal cortex in the vicinity of principal sulcus in an awake *M. mulatta*.[13] How does one know what the neuron records into memory? "The question naturally arises as to the character of the prefrontal contribution [to memory] compared to that of other areas [including, but not limited to hippocampus] and how it differs from these other areas" (Goldman-Rakic et al., 1990).

She doesn't assume that, *a priori*, a prefrontal neuron serves either memory or perception.

Unlike in sensory physiology, a prefrontal neuron's response recorded by a microelectrode isn't a function of some stimulus in the environment. More abstractly, its "memory field," akin yet different to a sensory receptive field, *isn't* immediately present in the environment. An external stimulus leads to execution of a response in trained monkeys, but there's a delay between the stimulus and a prompt for execution:

> The simple expedient of introducing a time delay
> forces the monkey to guide its response on the basis of an

---

[13] I don't mean to suggest that the study of prefrontal cortex described in this chapter involves only layer V pyramidal neurons. But Goldman-Rakic herself offers that layer V neurons hypothetically could be "presaccadic" (Goldman-Rakic et al., 1990).

internal representation, or memory, of the reward location. In the classic version of the task, after the monkey watches a reward being hidden under the cover of one of two food wells, an opaque screen is lowered to prevent the animal from reaching the hidden reward immediately. Following a 1-5 second delay, the screen is raised and selection of one of the locations is then allowed. Since the placement of the concealed item is randomly varied from trial to trial, the animal has to continually update his memory; accordingly, what is relevant on trial n becomes irrelevant on trial $n + 1$ (Goldman-Rakic et al., 1990).

The time frame of the delay is worth our notice. The subject's task is not to retain a long-term association for minutes or longer; the memory is more of the highly temporary, "working" variety. And: "It has been emphasized by cognitive theorists that working memory has at least two components–a storage component and a processing component" (Goldman-Rakic, 1995). We'll see an example of storage in a moment, but Goldman-Rakic observes that "[i]t is less easily shown that monkeys can process information, i.e., transform it mentally" (Goldman-Rakic, 1995). But her group will show that, too.

*

Storage. I'll simplify the oculomotor delayed-response task she used with her animals and will describe just three results, among many, from Funahashi et al., 1989.

A monkey has been trained to fix gaze on the lit center point of a screen, and does so for 0.75 of a second. Then a visual target is randomly presented in one of four eccentric locations–for example, 12-, 3-, 6-, and 9-o'clock positions on the screen. Let's say that the target appears at the 6 o'clock location for half a second, then disappears. The monkey maintains fixation at center point for that half second, then for a delay period lasting as long as five seconds. Once the lit center point vanishes, the monkey is supposed to make a visual saccade to the previously indicated 6 o'clock location within half a second.   Recording cylinders pass through the skull for the purpose of microelectrode recording of prefrontal neurons (recordings took place over the course of months); eye movements are measured by means of a coil implanted under the conjunctiva of one eye.

I'll discuss only neurons in the vicinity of principal sulcus, and should mention as well that they're specifically not neurons of the frontal eye field, which was studied separately.

In this next diagram, the central fixation point should be very much smaller than the target. But the protocol's steps are the interest:

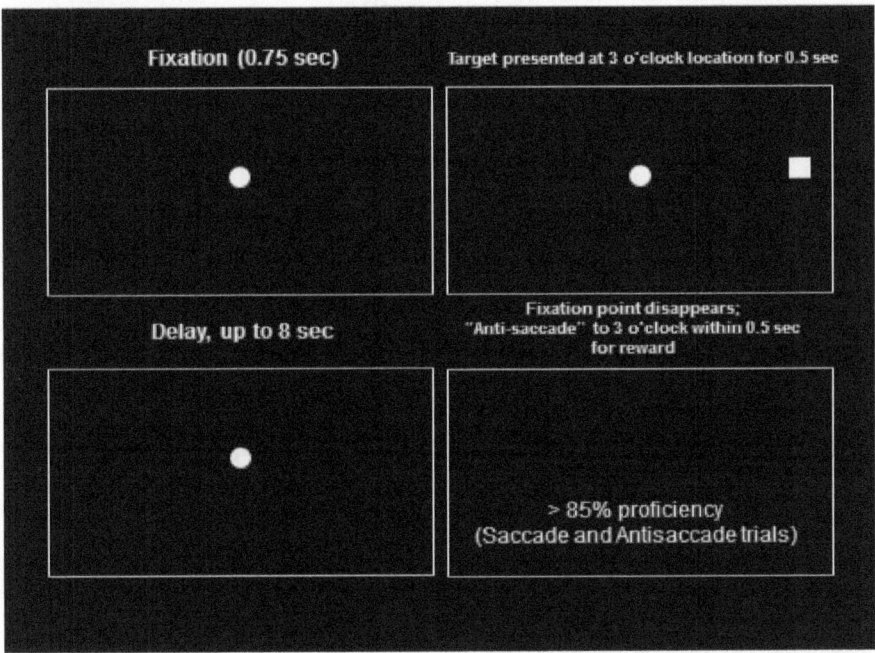

Result one: many, *not all*, principal sulcus neurons showed significantly increased firing rates compared to their baseline rates during the delay period for *at least one target location.*

Result two: in the case of one neuron used as an illustrative instance ("5211, left hemisphere"), its delay-period firing rate increased above baseline *only* if the target had been presented at 6 o'clock. And the firing rate decreased *below* baseline if the target had previously been presented at 12 o'clock.

Result three: when the "best directions" for entire samples of neurons were plotted in the aggregate for a given hemisphere, "there was a bias for representing the contralateral visual field in memory" (Goldman-Rakic, 1990).[14]

Thinking just about neuron 5211, its firing above baseline is specific for the 6 o'clock location if the target had been presented there, and its firing is inhibited if the target's prior location was at 12 o'clock. The firing doesn't cause the saccade.

Speaking anthropomorphically (always a danger, but here an unavoidable surmise), neuron 5211 remembers (stores) a position in space. Its firing is also inhibited if the preceding stimulus is presented in the upper, not lower, visual field.

*

Processing. In a variation on the protocol just described, monkeys were trained in a new "anti-saccade" task (Funahashi et al., 1993a):

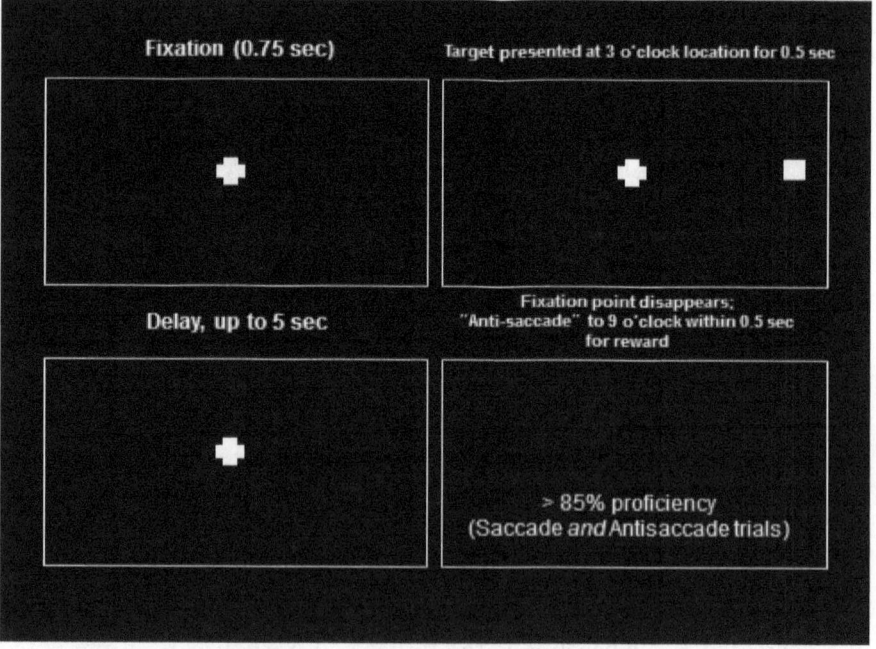

---

[14]   Corroboration for "sidedness" in memory can be found in Funahashi et al., 1993.

"The anti-saccade paradigm required the monkeys to suppress the automatic or prepotent ["prepotent" has to be Funahashi's word, used elsewhere in his own writing] tendency to respond in the direction of the remembered cue and instead respond in the opposite direction, a transformation that is not particularly easy for human subjects" (Goldman-Rakic, 1995). The same neurons were studied during saccade and anti-saccade sessions (Funahashi et al., 1993a).

*

Let's examine a single prefrontal neuron, say in left hemisphere, during either paradigm.

1. In the basic saccade task, a target presented in right visual hemispace elicits increased firing during the delay period. (Position preference led to the choice of the particular neuron to discuss.) A saccade successfully occurs to the 3 o'clock position.
2. In the anti-saccade task, a target presented in right visual hemispace elicits increased firing during the delay period. An anti-saccade successfully occurs to the *9 o'clock* position.
3. In the anti-saccade task, if the target is presented in *left* visual hemispace, firing rate of the left hemispheric neuron doesn't increase over baseline. Nevertheless, an anti-saccade successfully occurs to the 3 o'clock position.

The same neuron is studied. The "working" information remains the same—that is, increased firing during the delay period occurs independently of the task. But the tasks differ, with similar success rates for both saccades and anti-saccades during a session. The surmise is: it's *as if* the monkey processes prefrontal information to accomplish either task:

> . . . the same neuron involved in commanding an oculomotor response is also engaged when this response is suppressed and/or redirected. Such findings argue for at least a rudimentary form of propositional thinking on the part of nonhuman primates as well as point toward a cellular basis for mental processing in the nonhuman primate prefrontal cortex (Goldman-Rakic, 1995).

*

Noticing that F.A.H., J.VN., and R.W.G. were all about to speak after having listened to her with the ardor of those discovering novelty,[15] she took a short breath then said, "But there's one other thing."

---

[15] In this chapter and the next I review work from Goldman-Rakic's lab done as long as 35 years ago. Funahashi nicely discusses developments since his time in her lab, years after his return from the United States to Japan (Funahashi, 2017).

13

The Other Thing

. . ., she said, has to do with thalamus, about which we have heard a bit.

*

I think the best way to proceed, since I've already shared with the group at length, is to show and tell, she said. As you know, my lab has studied *M. mulatta*. For the sake of simplicity, I'll show you images of a different monkey's brain, that of the owl monkey or *Aotus trivirgatus*. *Aotus*'s cortex is less convoluted than *M. mulatta*'s, and I can make my points more clearly with simpler anatomy.

Consider a coronal section through prefrontal cortex (to the left, below). We had reason to believe that areas of circumferential prefrontal cortex at that level should receive afferents from medial dorsal nucleus of thalamus in the same hemisphere (the owl-monkey nucleus is circled to the right). If I may say so, it took nontrivial neurosurgical skill, but it was possible for us to place retrograde tracers throughout prefrontal cortex. The animals were alive at the time of surgery, but were sacrificed two days later (the time needed for tracer to pass from injection sites). We implanted in more than six places, but you'll get the idea of what we found in the series of pictures I've created for the group.

Let me say that I'm not sure what to make of what we found. Yet I find that there's an elegance to all of it (Goldman-Rakic and Porrino, 1985).

First, the coronal sections:

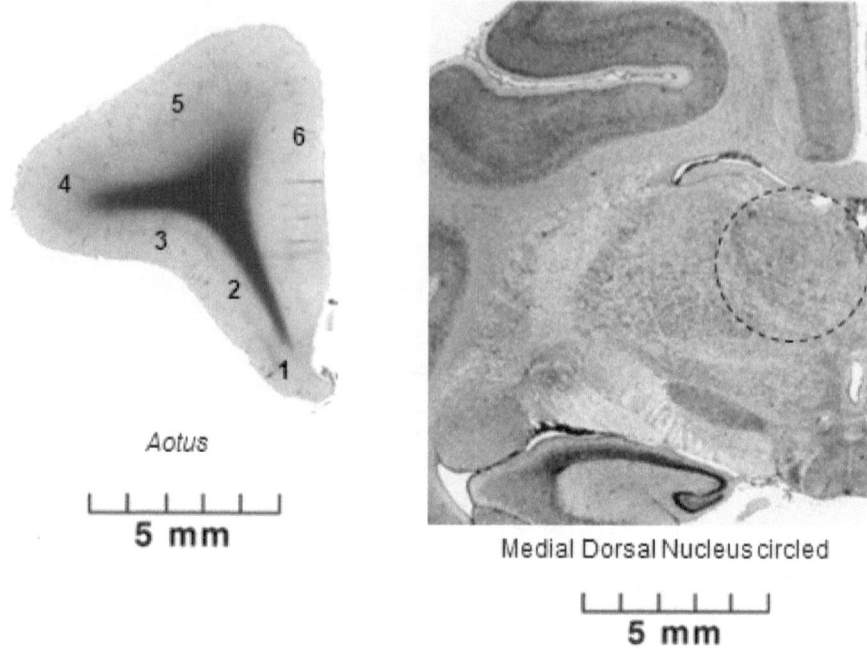

Aotus

5 mm

Medial Dorsal Nucleus circled

5 mm

Remember that a retrograde tracer works to visualize those places that *project to* the injection site. I indicate, schematically, two locations within medial dorsal nucleus associated with injection sites 1 and 3:

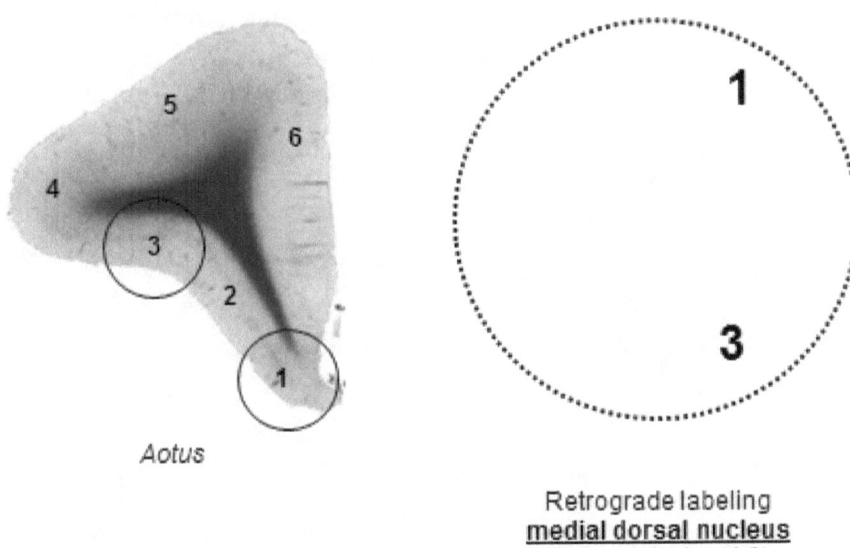

Aotus

Retrograde labeling
medial dorsal nucleus
(lesion site **1 and 3**)

Do you notice something about the order of the numbers? In prefrontal cortex, I've numbered in a counterclockwise fashion. In medial dorsal nucleus, we found labels organizing themselves in a clockwise direction, as you can see with all the sites now represented:

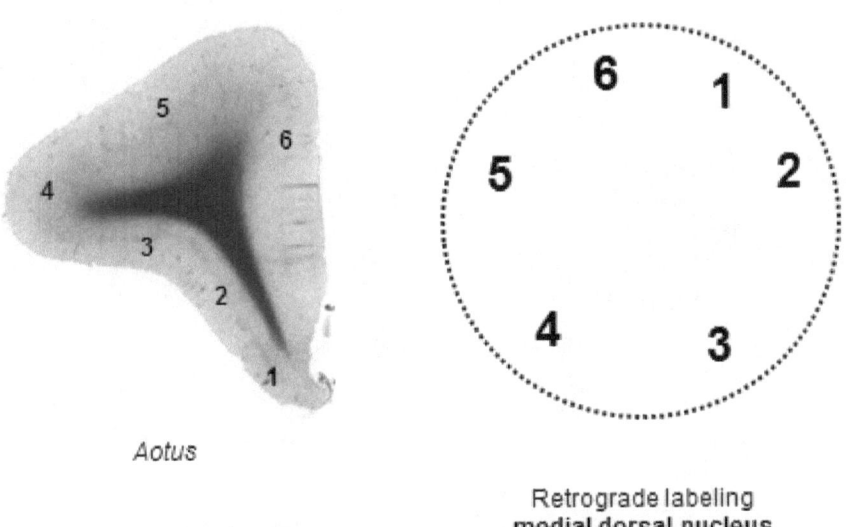

Aotus

Retrograde labeling
medial dorsal nucleus
(**ALL** lesion sites)

Two interesting twists follow. Retrograde labeling showed up elsewhere, notably in anterior nucleus of thalamus and medial pulvinar, though the order of the numbers varied between those discrete thalamic nuclei:

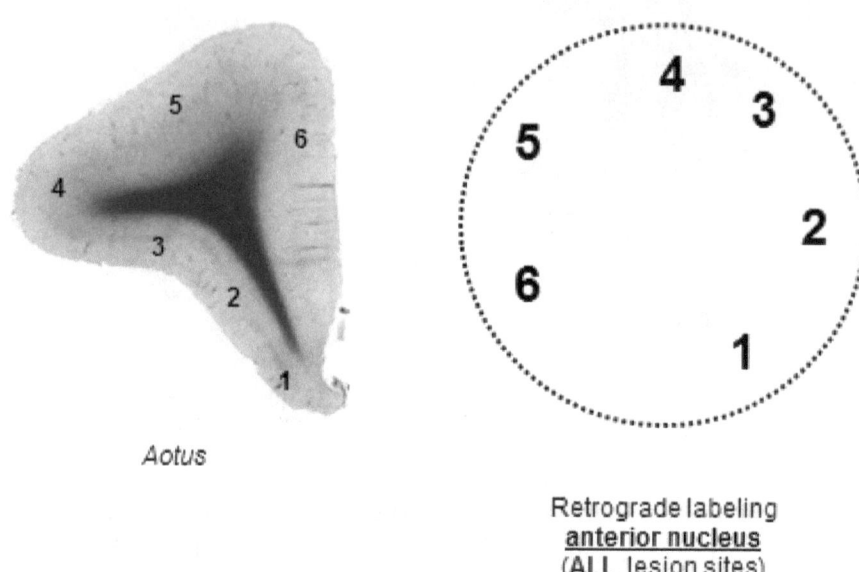

Aotus

Retrograde labeling
anterior nucleus
(ALL lesion sites)

And, in medial pulvinar, we found:

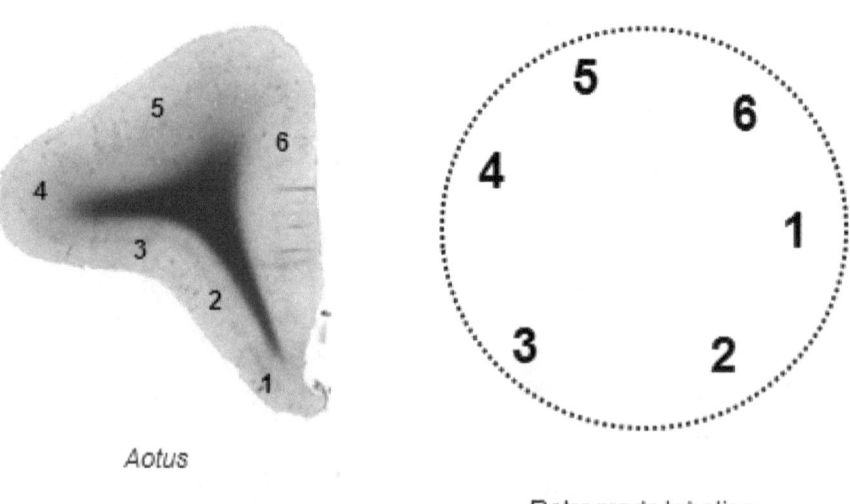

Aotus

Retrograde labeling
medial pulvinar nucleus
(ALL lesion sites)

We have no doubt that occipital cortex and frontal cortex are linked to each other, not only via thalamus, but also by fibers "of association," as they're called.

But we think it's reasonable to conclude that prefrontal cortex can be defined by choreographed relations with multiple thalamic locales.[16]

*

How very analog, J.V.N. said. The diagrams look like a rotary phone dial of a bygone time. A rotary phone dial in various moments of its use, I should say.

Anterior, medial dorsal, and pulvinar nuclei are higher order, R.W.G. said.

Nihil est intellectu quod non antea fuerit in sensu, F.A.H. said.[17]

---

[16] For an *anterograde* labeling study, see Selemon and Goldman-Rakic, 1988, a paper that corroborates a notion of a distributed mnemonic/prefrontal network involved, at least, in some types of sensory based memory.

[17] The Latin sentence is John Locke's maxim of empiricism, quoted in Hayek, 1994. *Nothing is in the mind which is not placed there by the senses.* Locke, we tend to forget, given his stature as a philosopher, studied medicine.

PART IV

14

Tabulated Nuclei, Graphed Connectivity

A book named *Thalamus and Its Cortex* would have to include some summary of parts of thalamus in relationship to cortical areas and, while we're at it, an overview of other inputs and outputs to and from thalamus. There have been many textbook attempts—we'll study examples. In light of the preceding chapter, there's reasonable doubt that any summary can do justice to the subtleties involved for all nuclei. There are other cautions to consider, not least of which is whether studies in non-human animals translate to the human brain.[18]

Nevertheless, we can specify our procedure and proceed: 1. Start with five instances of input and output summaries of thalamocortex[19]; 2. Abide by Jones's nomenclature of thalamic nuclei, summarized below; 3. Attempt specificity regarding cortical areas whenever possible (a "diffuse" thalamic

---

[18] For example, Kass and Baldwin (2020) discuss how a temporal lobe area such as primate "area MT" in the dorsal visual stream or a pulvinar nucleus, each activated powerfully by superior colliculus, *isn't* found in "tree shrews or rodents, and likely any other [non-primate] mammals."

[19] Sources off the shelf are: Carpenter and Sutin, 1983; Jones, 1985; Nieuwenhuys et al., 2008; Nolte, 1999; Sherman and Koch, 1998. The choices are personal. There have been other summaries based on new research modalities in animals (papers cited in what follows) and based on human functional imaging (e.g., Zhang et al., 2010).

---

projection is a vagary that we'll avoid); 4. Stick to nuclei of the parent list without division of nuclear groups (e.g., the several nuclei associated with anterior nuclear group or the two habenular nuclei; the exception will be pulvinar, which we divide just into two parts); 5. Concentrate on nuclei that we've either seen or mentioned in our preceding chapters; 6. For each nucleus, choose recent papers using novel methods and contemporary reviews to identify or corroborate connections, and include their findings; 7. Collate what all the sources report.

*

Parent List, with abbreviations (modified from Jones, 1985)

A	Anterior nuclear group
CeM	*Centre médian* nucleus (an intralaminar nucleus)
H	Habenula
LD	Lateral dorsal nucleus
LGN	Lateral geniculate nucleus (not the "complex" that includes pregeniculate nucleus, among others)
LP	Lateral posterior nuclear complex
MD	Medial dorsal nucleus
MGN	Medial geniculate nucleus (not the "complex" responsible for projections beyond primary auditory cortex)
Para	Paraventricular nucleus of thalamus
Pf	Parafascicular nucleus (an intralaminar nucleus)
Pll	Pulvinar, lateral
Plm	Pulvinar, medial
Po	Posterior nuclear complex
Pt	Parataenial nucleus
R	Reticular nucleus
VA, VL	Ventral anterior nucleus and Ventral lateral nucleus considered together
VM	Ventral medial nuclear group
VP	Ventral posterior nucleus (medial VP [**VPM**] and lateral VP [**VPL**] considered together)

*

A: anterior nuclear group

Subcortical input	Subcortical output	Cortical output	Cortical input
mammillary bodies via mammillothalamic tract; ascending noradrenergic and cholinergic brainstem projections (Jones, p. 697); hypothalamus and pretectum (Jones, pp. 686-694); Perry and Mitchell, 2019 add midbrain tegmentum; (see **R**)	habenula (**H**) via *stria medullaris* (described by some investigators per Carpenter and Sutin, p. 506); (see **R**)	**cingulate gyrus;** subiculum[20]; presubiculum; parasubiculum; **retrosplenial cortex** (Thompson and Robertson, 1987); primary olfactory cortex per Sherman and Koch; **entorhinal cortex** (O'Mara and Aggleton, 2019); Zhang et al., 2010 corroborate cingulate and retrosplenial projections. Hunnicutt et al., 2014 add "infralimbic [medial frontal] cortex" in the rat, medial orbital, and motor cortex. Perry and Mitchell, 2019 add temporal association cortex, visual areas V1 and V2, and secondary (S2) sensory cortex.	*reciprocal*: **cingulate gyrus;** presubiculum; parasubiculum; **retrosplenial cortex; entorhinal cortex;** hippocampus via **postcommissural fornix** Prasad et al., 2020: primary sensory cortex and medial prefrontal cortex

---

[20] For a discussion of subiculum and other subicular structures in their relationship to entorhinal cortex, see *Teaching Hippocampal Anatomy*.

CeM: *centre médian* nucleus (see also Pf)

Subcortical input	Subcortical output	Cortical output	Cortical input
medial *globus pallidus*; spinothalamic fibers of spinal cord; reticular formation; parabrachial nucleus of pons; per Smith et al., 2009: *locus ceruleus*, dorsal *raphe* nuclei, cholinergic nuclei (e.g., pedunculopontine nucleus, part of a **"mesencephalic locomotor region"** [Sébille et al., 2017]); deep layers of superior colliculus; pretectum; supramammillary area (hypothalamus) per Van der Werf et al., 2002; *substantia nigra pars reticulata*; deep cerebellar nuclei; also, per Thompson and Robertson, 1987, nucleus of diagonal band of Broca; (see **R**)	*corpus striatum*; In squirrel monkeys, per Van der Werf et al., 2002: globus pallidus (internal and external segments), nucleus of *tractus solitarius*, *substantia nigra pars reticulata*. (see **R**)	**primary motor cortex**; elsewhere in frontal lobe; parietal lobe; Cortical projections from intralaminar nuclei might represent collaterals of thalamostriate fibers, per Carpenter and Sutin. But: Van der Werf et al., 2002 specifically cite terminal labeling (anterograde tracer) of dorsolateral frontal and parietal cortices, including primary sensory cortex.	*reciprocal*: **primary motor cortex** ("massive," per Carpenter and Sutin, p. 512); elsewhere in frontal lobe Prasad et al., 2020: primary motor cortex and medial prefrontal cortex

H: habenula (epithalamic, not technically part of dorsal thalamus); see Hikosaka, 2010

Subcortical input	Subcortical output	Cortical output	Cortical input
septum via *stria medullaris*; diagonal band of Broca; *nucleus basalis* of Meynert; lateral hypothalamus; lateral preoptic area; medial *globus pallidus*	via **habenulo-peduncular tract** (*fasciculus retroflexus*): interpeduncular nucleus (subsequently, midbrain *raphe* nuclei); midbrain tegmental nuclei; *substantia nigra pars compacta* bilaterally; ventral tegmental area; hypothalamus bilaterally	*Indirect* cortical effects via dopamine, other neurotransmitters	bilateral prepiriform cortex; medial frontal cortex Prasad et al., 2020 corroborate medial prefrontal cortex

LD: lateral dorsal nucleus (compare to **A**)

Subcortical input	Subcortical output	Cortical output	Cortical input
pretectum (retinal-recipient and non-retinal recipient); no evidence for a projection from mammillary bodies (see Jones, p. 693 and Nieuwenhuys et al., p. 264); Perry and Mitchell, 2019 add superior colliculus and **LGN**. (see **R**)	mammillary bodies (part of a "lateral head direction circuit"–see Perry and Mitchell, 2019); (see **R**)	**cingulate gyrus;** subiculum, presubiculum, parasubiculum; retrosplenial cortex; **entorhinal cortex** (O'Mara and Aggleton, 2019); Hunnicutt et al., 2014 add motor cortices (M1, M2), primary sensory cortex and primary visual cortex; Perry and Mitchell, 2019 add secondary (S2) sensory and visual area V2.	*reciprocal*: **cingulate gyrus;** presubiculum, parasubiculum; retrosplenial cortex; **entorhinal cortex;** hippocampus via postcommissural fornix; inferior parietal lobule per Carpenter and Sutin, p. 514 Prasad et al., 2020: primary sensory cortex, primary visual cortex, primary motor cortex

LGN: lateral geniculate nucleus

Subcortical input	Subcortical output	Cortical output	Cortical input
optic tract from **retina**; superior colliculus; Nakamura, 2018 adds deep cerebellar nuclei; (see **R**)	superior colliculus; **LP**; (See Monavarfeshani et al., 2017 and Nakamura, 2018 for discussion of other subcortical inputs and outputs, including output to thalamic nuclei other than **LP** and **R**; also to suprachiasmatic nucleus of hypothalamus, pineal gland, and pretectum.) (see **R**)	**primary visual cortex**	*reciprocal*: **primary visual cortex**

LP: lateral posterior nuclear complex (see also **Plm** and **Pll**)

Subcortical input	Subcortical output	Cortical output	Cortical input
superior colliculus; Nieuwenhuys et al., p. 266 add pretectum; ?from **VP** per Carpenter and Sutin, p. 514; other neighboring nuclei; retina, per Jones, p. 553; (see **R**)	?to **VP**, other neighboring nuclei; (see **R**)	**superior and inferior parietal lobules** per Carpenter and Sutin, p. 514 and Impieri et al., 2018; "posterior parietal lobe" per Mayer et al., 2019; areas 17 (**primary visual cortex**) and 18 (~**V2**), perisylvian cortex in cats per Jones, p. 548; primary and V2 cortex in mice and cingulate gyrus (Hu et al., 2019); primary and secondary motor and sensory cortices and (to a lesser degree) retrosplenial cortex per Hunnicutt et al., 2014	*reciprocal*: **superior and inferior parietal lobules**; **areas 17 and 18**, ?perisylvian cortex; Hu et al. (2019) add cingulate gyrus to anterior portions of **LP**.

MD: medial dorsal nucleus

Subcortical input	Subcortical output	Cortical output	Cortical input
amygdala via bed nuclei of the *stria terminalis* per Nieuwenhuys et al., p.264; *substantia nigra pars reticulata*; ventral *globus pallidus*, per Carpenter and Sutin, p. 507;	likely reciprocal with **CeM**, other intralaminar nuclei, lateral thalamic nuclei; Kuramoto et al., 2017 identify a reciprocal connection to and from **neostriatum**.	**prefrontal cortex; olfactory and limbic structures;** Zhang et al., 2010 specify frontal eye field, orbitofrontal, medial and lateral frontal cortices;	*reciprocal*: **prefrontal cortex; olfactory and limbic structures** (entorhinal and perirhinal cortices and cortex of the temporal pole, per Nieuwenhuys et al., p. 264.
CeM; other intralaminar nuclei; lateral thalamic nuclei; superior colliculus; pretectum; vestibular nuclei; midbrain tegmentum;	(see **R**)	Hunnicutt et al., 2014 and Alcaraz et al., 2016 cite ventral, medial orbital prefrontal cortices, but Hunnicutt et al. add insula, and M2 motor cortex.	Stepniewska et al., 2007 cite sparse projections from premotor cortex. Vertes et al., 2015 add entorhinal cortex
Vertes et al., 2015 add *nucleus accumbens septi*, medial *globus pallidus*, hypothalamus, diagonal band of Broca, reticular formation, ventral tegmental area, *substantia nigra pars compacta, locus ceruleus, raphe* nuclei		Kuramoto et al., 2017 report: "The main target areas of MD neurons were the prefrontal, secondary motor, and frontal association areas, and additionally MD neurons sent a small number of	Prasad et al., 2020: primary sensory cortex, primary motor cortex, medial prefrontal cortex
Çavdar et al. 2014 add deep cerebellar nuclei (dentate) and *zona incerta*.		axon fibers, less than 30 mm in axon length, to the primary motor, secondary visual, and retrosplenial areas."	
(see **R**)			

MGN: medial geniculate nucleus

Subcortical input	Subcortical output	Cortical output	Cortical input
lateral lemniscus via brachium of inferior colliculus; **(see R)**	Jones, pp. 434-439, warns that we shouldn't undersell the tripartite division of the medial geniculate *complex* (and the complex's connections with inferior colliculus) in species such as the cat, tree shrew, and monkey. (see **R**)	**primary auditory cortex**	*reciprocal*: **primary auditory cortex**

Para: paraventricular nucleus of thalamus (epithalamic, not technically part of dorsal thalamus)

Subcortical input	Subcortical output	Cortical output	Cortical input
preoptic area; hypothalamus; Van der Werf et al., 2002 cite tuberomammillary nucleus (histaminergic in hypothalamus), ventral tegmental area, *locus ceruleus, raphe* nuclei, nucleus of *tractus solitarius*, parabrachial nucleus (dorsal pons), bed nuclei of *stria terminalis*, amygdala; Salazar-Juárez et al., 2002 describe reciprocal connection with suprachiasmatic nucleus; Nascimento et al., 2008 describe a direct retinal input in a rodent species;	?reciprocal with preoptic area; hypothalamus (suprachiasmatic nucleus, lateral hypothalamus); claustrum; septum; ***nucleus accumbens septi/*"extended amygdala"/ amygdala** (Otis et al., 2019; Parsons et al., 2007; Abivardi and Bach, 2017); nucleus of diagonal band of Broca (Heredia et al., 2002); periaqueductal grey; (ventrolateral) medulla per Ogundele et al., 2017	medial prefrontal cortex, insula, subiculum per Vertes et al. 2015	medial prefrontal cortex and insula per Vertes et al., 2015; Van der Werf et al., 2002 add subiculum Prasad et al., 2020 and Otis et al., 2019: medial prefrontal cortex

Otis et al., 2019 discuss lateral hypothalamus (see also Hsu and Price, 2009); septum and periaqueductal grey (see Heredia et al., 2002); per Thompson and Robertson, 1987, nucleus of diagonal band of Broca; Vertes et al., 2015 add midbrain nuclei, both pretectal and tegmental.			

Pf: parafascicular nucleus (see also CeM)

Subcortical input	Subcortical output	Cortical output	Cortical input
putamen; **deep cerebellar nuclei;** *nucleus accumbens septi;* medial *globus pallidus;* ?periaqueductal grey; **"mesencephalic locomotor region"** (includes pedunculopontine nucleus) (Sébille et al., 2017); spinothalamic fibers of spinal cord (see **CeM**); Van der Werf et al., 2002 add *substantia nigra pars reticulata, zona incerta*, pretectum, deep cerebellar nuclei, reticular formation (including indoleamine and catecholamine nuclei), parabrachial nucleus (dorsal pons), nucleus of the solitary tract, medulla (several nuclei), vestibular nuclei. (see **R**)	*corpus striatum;* There's debate, based on studies dating to the 1950's, about whether **Pf** projects mainly to caudate, putamen, or *nucleus accumbens septi* as discussed by Jones, p. 626. Van der Werf et al., 2002 add *nucleus basalis* of Meynert and *substantia innominata,* subthalamic nucleus, reticular formation, nucleus of the solitary tract, inferior olive, hypothalamus; and, in squirrel moneys, *globus pallidus, substantia nigra pars reticulata*, and ventral tegmental area. Lee et al., 2020 specifically report reciprocal connection to and from ***substantia nigra pars reticulata.*** (see **R**)	**frontal, medial, dorsolateral cortex;** perhaps to as far as the occiput; Cortical projections from intralaminar nuclei might represent collaterals of thalamostriate fibers, per Carpenter and Sutin. But: Van der Werf et al., 2002 cite terminal labeling (anterograde tracer) of dorsal and lateral frontal and parietal cortices. Mandelbaum et al., 2019 are more specific: cingulate, insula, limbic/medial frontal cortex (viz., infra- and prelimbic areas in the mouse), primary motor cortex, primary and secondary sensory cortex.	*reciprocal*: **frontal, medial, dorsolateral cortex**, at least Prasad et al., 2020: primary motor cortex, primary sensory cortex

Pll: pulvinar, lateral (see also **Plm**)

Subcortical input	Subcortical output	Cortical output	Cortical input
superior colliculus; pretectum; ?from retina directly; (see **R**)	-- Corticotectal fibers traverse **Pll**, but Carpenter and Sutin call those fibers extensions of the external medullary lamina of thalamus. (see **R**)	parietotemporal cortex; "posterior parietal lobe" per Mayer et al., 2019; Impieri et al., 2018 discuss superior parietal lobule; **occipital cortex; multiple visual areas of the ventral stream**, e.g., V4 cortex (Zhou et al., 2016)	*reciprocal*: parietotemporal cortex; **occipital cortex; visual areas of the ventral stream** Prasad et al., 2020: primary sensory cortex, primary visual cortex

Plm: pulvinar, medial (see also Pll)

Subcortical input	Subcortical output	Cortical output	Cortical input
superior colliculus; ?pretectum Jones isn't convinced about collicular and pretectal input to either **Pll** or **Plm**; note that there's also an *inferior* part to **Pl**, which clearly receives from superior colliculus and pretectum, per Jones, p. 551. Nieuwenhuys et al., p. 266, identify projections "from deep, non-visual layers" of superior colliculus specifically to **Plm.** (see **R**)	?amygdala, per Jones, pp. 560-561; (see **R**)	**superior temporal gyrus; prefrontal cortex;** Impieri et al., 2018 discuss superior parietal lobule; Zhang et al. (2010) adds parietotemporal and occipital cortices; "posterior parietal lobe" per Mayer et al., 2019	*reciprocal*: **superior temporal gyrus; prefrontal cortex** Prasad et al., 2020: primary sensory cortex, primary visual cortex

Po: posterior nuclear complex

Subcortical input	Subcortical output	Cortical output	Cortical input
afferents related to noxious stimuli–?in particular: spinothalamic, lemniscal, and cervicothalamic fibers of spinal cord per Jones, p. 589; superior colliculus; inferior colliculus; (see **R**)	Lateral **Po** has been regarded *as part of* both anterior **MGN** and **VP**, per Jones, p. 585); (see **R**)	**insula; retroinsular cortex** surrounding secondary sensory cortex; frontal association, primary and secondary motor and sensory cortices per Hunnicutt et al., 2014; primary motor cortex per Mo and Sherman, 2019	*reciprocal*: **insula; retroinsular cortex** surrounding secondary sensory cortex primary sensory cortex and auditory cortex per Carpenter and Sutin, p. 523 Prasad et al., 2020: primary motor cortex

Pt: parataenial nucleus

Subcortical input	Subcortical output	Cortical output	Cortical input
nucleus accumbens septi; claustrum (O'Mara and Aggleton, 2019); (see **R**)	*nucleus accumbens septi*; claustrum and ventral *corpus striatum* per Van der Werf et al., 2002; (see **R**)	?*taenia tecta* (ventral medial frontal lobe, near *n. accumbens*); "infralimbic" and "prelimbic" cortex (medial frontal), subiculum per Van der Werf et al., 2002; medial orbitofrontal cortex and "infralimbic cortex" (medial frontal) per Hunnicutt et al., 2014); subiculum (Jankowski et al., 2015 and O'Mara and Aggleton, 2019)	***reciprocal***: subiculum Prasad et al., 2020: medial prefrontal cortex

R: reticular nucleus (part of "ventral," not "dorsal" thalamus)

Subcortical input	Subcortical output	Cortical output	Cortical input
midbrain tegmentum; **all dorsal thalamic nuclei**	**all dorsal thalamic nuclei**	_none_	**all areas of cortex** Prasad et al., 2020: primary sensory cortex, primary motor cortex, medial prefrontal cortex

VA, VL: ventral anterior nucleus and ventral lateral nucleus considered together

Subcortical input	Subcortical output	Cortical output	Cortical input
medial *globus pallidus*; **contralateral deep cerebellar nuclei;** *substantia nigra pars reticulata*; part of spinothalamic tract, per Jones, pp. 396-399; vestibular nuclei per Jones, pp. 399-403; intralaminar and midline thalamic nuclei; (see **R**)	intralaminar nuclei; **MD;** (see **R**)	**precentral frontal cortex;** Zhang et al., 2010 adds cingulate gyrus; Stepniewska et al., 2007 corroborate "dense" projection to premotor areas; Impieri et al., 2018 discuss superior parietal lobule; Hunnicutt et al., 2014 cite frontal association, primary and secondary motor cortices and, to a lesser degree, retrosplenial cortex.	*reciprocal*: **precentral frontal cortex** Prasad et al., 2020: primary sensory cortex, primary motor cortex, medial prefrontal cortex

VM: ventral medial nuclear group

Subcortical input	Subcortical output	Cortical output	Cortical input
substantia nigra pars reticulata; spinothalamic tract and trigeminothalamic projection; **nucleus of solitary tract** (taste related) per Jones, pp. 418-423; dorsal pontine parabrachial nucleus (taste related); caudal medulla per Jones, pp. 418-423; (see **R**)	overlap with **VP** (**VPM**); Lee et al., 2020 specifically report reciprocal connection to and from *substantia nigra pars reticulata*. (see **R**)	**insula**; prefrontal cortex; **primary sensory cortex**; Stepniewska et al., 2007 cite some (less-than-dense) projections to premotor areas; Guo et al., 2018 add primary motor cortex, as does Hunnicutt et al., 2014.	*reciprocal*: **insula**; ?prefrontal cortex; **primary sensory cortex** Prasad et al., 2020: primary sensory cortex, primary motor cortex, medial prefrontal cortex

VP: ventral posterior nucleus (medial VP [VPM] and lateral VP [VPL] considered together)

Subcortical input	Subcortical output	Cortical output	Cortical input
medial and trigeminal lemnisci; spinothalamic tract (spinal cord); central tegmental tract conveying taste information (from nucleus of solitary tract) per Nolte, p. 389; (see **R**)	Lateral **Po** has been regarded *as part of* **VP** per Jones, p. 585. (see **R**)	**primary and secondary sensory cortices;** Hunnicutt et al., 2014 add motor cortices (mainly primary motor cortex); Impieri et al., 2018 discuss superior parietal lobule.	*reciprocal*: **primary and secondary sensory cortices** Prasad et al., 2020: primary sensory cortex, primary motor cortex

*

The above tables aren't the only way to depict the information within them. As a next step, let's first provide legends for abbreviations in presentations that follow.

Alphabetically, here are subcortical sites that project to thalamic nuclei, based on our review:

Amyg: amygdala; **Bed**: bed nuclei of *stria terminalis*; **C**: spinal cord; **Cl**: claustrum; **CM**: caudal medulla; **DBB**: diagonal band of Broca; **DCN**: deep cerebellar nuclei; **GPi/VGP**: internal (or medial) *globus pallidus* and ventral *globus pallidus*; **Hyp**: hypothalamus; **IC**: inferior colliculus; **IC(b)**: brachium of inferior colliculus; **IO**: inferior olive; **LH**: lateral hypothalamus; **LPO**: lateral preoptic area; **Med**: medulla (e.g., ventrolateral medulla); **MB**: mammillary bodies; **MTg**: midbrain tegmentum; **MLR**: mesencephalic locomotor region (per Sébille et al., 2017); **NAS**: *nucleus accumbens septi*; **NB**: *nucleus basalis*; **NE/Ach/5HT**: brainstem nuclei related to norepinephprine, acetylcholine, serotonin; **NST**: nucleus of the solitary tract; **PAG**: periaqueductal grey; **POA**: preoptic area; **PPn**: (dorsal) pontine parabrachial nucleus; **PrT**: pretectum; **Put**: putamen; **RET**: retina; **RF**: reticular formation; **SC**: superior colliculus; **Sept**: septum; **SNpc**: substantia nigra pars compacta; **SNpr**: *substantia nigra pars reticulata*; **Str**: (corpus) striatum; **Vnn**: vestibular nuclei; **VTA**: ventral tegmental area; **ZI**: *zona incerta*.

And here are cited cortical areas that receive projections from thalamic nuclei:

A1: primary auditory cortex; **Cing**: cingulate gyrus; **dlPF**: dorsolateral prefrontal cortex; **ent**: entorhinal cortex; **"F"**: frontal cortex; **ins**: insula; **"L/H"**: limbic cortex/hippocampus; **M1**: primary motor cortex; **M2**: secondary motor cortex; **mPF**: medial prefrontal cortex; **"O"**: occipital cortex; **Olf1**: primary olfactory cortex; **"P"**: parietal lobe; **parasub**: parasubiculum; **presub**: presubiculum; **"PF"**: prefrontal cortex; **"PT"**: parieto-temporal cortex; **retroins**: retroinsular cortex; **retrosplen**: retrosplenial cortex; **S1**: primary sensory cortex; **S2**: secondary sensory cortex; **S/IPL**: superior and inferior parietal lobules; **STG**: superior temporal gyrus; **sub**: subiculum; **V1**: primary visual cortex; **V2**: area V2 (extrastriate visual cortex); **V4**: area V4 (ventral extrastriate visual cortex).

*

Visualizing subcortical projections to thalamus (thicker lines indicate first-order connections), there's a sense of *converging* input, not only to dorsal thalamic nuclei, but also to epithalamus (paraventricular nucleus of thalamus and habenula):

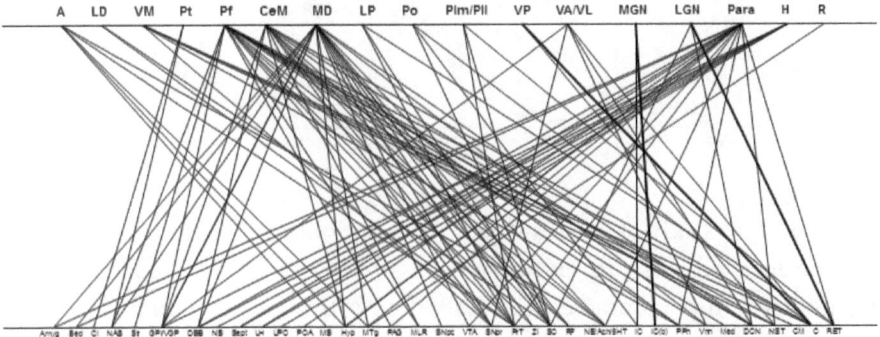

Looking at thalamic projections *to cortex*, one observes *diverging* output. Thicker lines again indicate relays from first-order nuclei (I include MGN as first order) which represent a minority of dorsal thalamic nuclei:

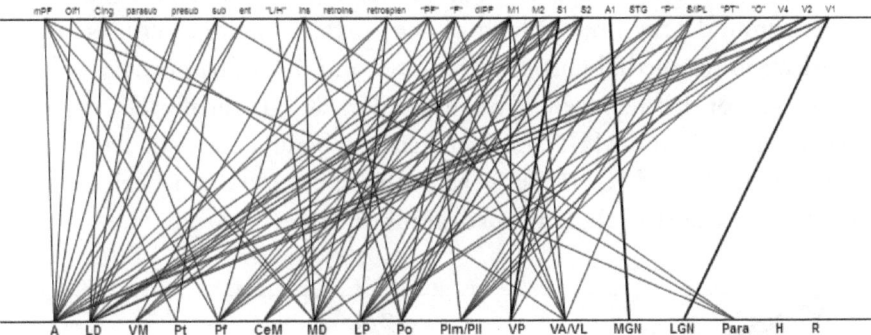

Anatomically anterior and medial thalamic nuclei dispatch an especially dense net across cortex:

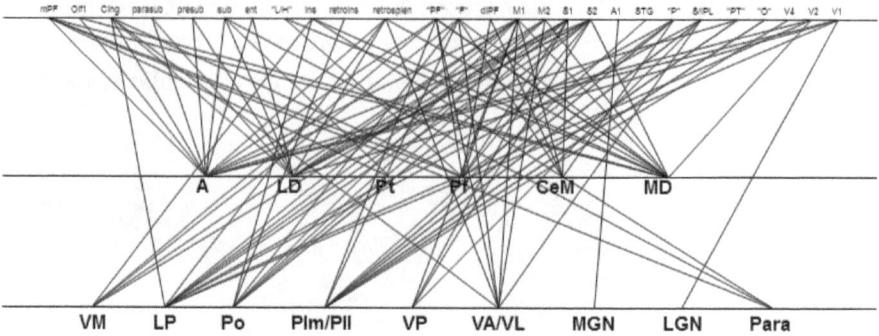

Based on study of cortical layer V projections to dorsal thalamus–and, as was learned, also to extrathalamic sites–after specific cortical areal injections in mice (Prasad et al., 2020), there's divergence in corticothalamic communication to counterpoint divergence in connections going the other way (from thalamus to cortex). Prasad et al.'s study interrogated only four cortical locales, but one observes that corticothalamic and thalamocortical projections are more than reciprocal. In the next figure, we indicate corticothalamic projections described by Prasad et al. with thick black lines. Thalamocortical projections illustrated previously are depicted as background grey lines. Much of the cortical mantle, perhaps with a predilection for medial cortical structures and, laterally, primary cortices (motor, sensory), is represented by twelve dorsal thalamic nuclei (putatively first-order LGN and MGN are excluded). Habenula and reticular nucleus of thalamus (**H** and **R**, respectively; both are of epithalamic origin) don't directly contribute to thalamocortical innervation

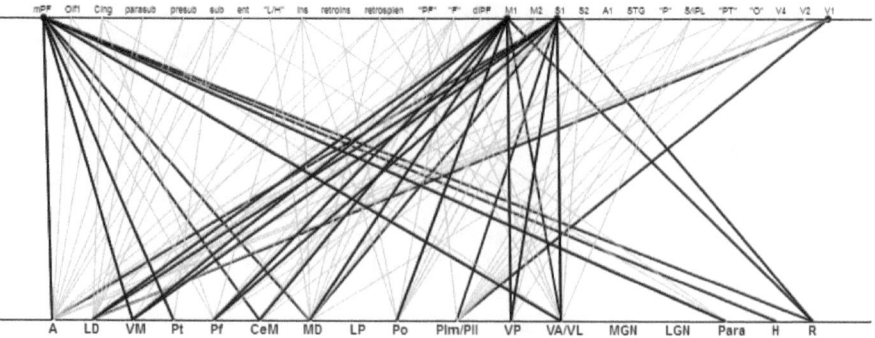

The limitation in the above images is that they don't provide a sense of the temporal progress among crisscrosses of connectivity–a situation analogous to a route map without representation of when planes or trains depart and arrive. In time-series graphs, precisely when point-to-point connections happen in time matters as much as the fact that the connections exist in the first place (for a discussion relevant to biology, see Douard, 1995 and Marey, 1885–in the latter, see pp. 19-22 in particular).

One can't disagree that functional and anatomic connections, as we currently understand them, underscore thalamus as a relay structure "that faithfully performs the duty of signal transmission" (Zhang et al., 2010). But the statement is only nominally correct. We observe that a.) anatomically anterior and medial thalamic nuclei evince a particularly wide net of connection with overlying cortex; and b.) medial cortex–including not only mesial temporal lobe, but also much of the parasagittal midline of the entire brain–and primary cortical domains (motor and sensory) in the lateral hemispheres are most densely represented by thalamocortical connectivity. Future study of thalamocortex shouldn't be weighted to a bias that the sole function served by thalamus is faithful signal transmission.[21]

The anatomy suggests the brain's afferentation is a function of changing convergence and bidirectional divergence of data streams across time.

---

[21] Nakajima and Halassa (2017) speak of the "well-recognized role of certain thalamic circuits in relaying categorical content," but that role differs from "control of connectivity within and across task-relevant [as opposed to content-bound] cortical networks."

15

Organizer's Commentary

Perhaps more so in a seminar than in other contexts, a classroom is where surprise happens. A teacher might have an idea about what should be accomplished, but actual proceedings can upend planning. When the unexpected happens, a class could be all the more interesting and memorable as a consequence. At any rate, such was the hope for this monograph's experiment in pedagogy.

Philosophical aspects (for lack of a better adjective) introduced in the first chapters yield to anatomy, which dominates all that follows. The purpose of the seminar has been to impart some anatomy, after all. Yet it's hard to overlook abstractions—notions of category and memory, for example—inherent in any discussion of sensory experience as mediated by thalamus.

As a result of exposure to Ernst Mach's (1838-1916) physiological psychology early in F.A.H.'s career, yet still quite originally when he wrote in the early 1950's, Hayek noticed a fallacy in thinking that sensory experience isn't abstract. Support for a notion that the senses are *higher* cortical functions comes from animal study—for example, ". . . fishes and birds that show that they respond in the same manner to a great variety of shapes which have only some very abstract features in common" (Hayek, 1978). He continues:

. . . probably most animals recognize, not what we would regard as concrete particulars, or particular individuals, but abstract features long before they can identify particulars. . . . Similar insights have been gained in human sensory psychology in the course of its gradual emancipation from the conception of simple elementary sensations from which, in a mosaic fashion, the representations of the environment were supposed to be built up.

The difference between a concrete particular and a representation, in Hayek's sense of both, is worth clarifying. He wouldn't and couldn't dispute that a visual representation happens as a result of neuronal processing based on very specific sensory receptive fields. He merely observes that no "concrete" detail (the sight of something centered on both foveae, for example) can be perceived in the absence of an abstract capacity to process information transmitted in the visual pathway. In other words, what isn't a representation in a brain?

On the subject of categories or classifications (A vs. B), we've mentioned a ball-selecting machine described in Hayek's *The Sensory Order* (1976). It's a strange device, but so too is the notion of a category of representation—I use "strange" in the sense of an unexpected goad to thought:

The classifications which the mind acquires to sort out undifferentiated sensations stem from prior experience. "Every sensation, even the 'purest' must therefore be regarded as an interpretation of an event in light of the past experience of the individual or the species." The use of a prior classification to determine the 'sense' of a sensation differs from . . . an a priori category in that Hayek's classifications emerge within the process of perception itself and *do not remain fixed*. They are not equivalent to a principle or axiom. (My emphasis, Hayek, 1994, p. 26.)

The issue is sensation as a function of time. In the passage, there's passing reference to the experience *of species*. That's quite a claim, to which we'll return in a bit. First, however, let's review where we've been in terms of individual sensory experience as a process.

Von Neumann, a mathematician and a pioneer of computer design, stipulates memory as an engineering requirement for any serial processing device, biological or otherwise. Are sensory systems working in real time *not* memory dependent? With Von Neumann, we'd say it's implausible.[22]

Two discussions needed to happen in light of that requirement, we felt. The first relates to the often-used term "efference copy" (it's used a lot in neuroscience, at least). Von Holst and Mittelstaedt's 1950 paper is still the best definition of the term; but R.W. Guillery's "Anatomical Pathways that Link Perception and Action" (2005) develops a thought, implicit in the definition, that past (and ongoing) motor activity and sensory corollary discharge are both parts of the "copy."

A second, even-more-necessary discussion centers on Goldman-Rakic's psychic cells of prefrontal cortex. Not surprisingly, her lab's work before her premature death occupies a big part of this monograph. Perhaps our book should be longer just to address more of her work. We've concentrated on information *presented just recently* in the sensory domain and on her lab's research regarding that particular mnemonic aspect.

In 1990, she wrote that delay-period firing wasn't exclusively a feature of prefrontal neurons, that similar discharge had been observed, by her lab and by others', in neurons of frontal eye field, posterior parietal cortex, premotor and motor cortices, hippocampus, and even basal ganglia (Goldman-Rakic et al., 1990). Maybe, she wondered, prefrontal delay activity had to do with rapid information processing (*just* on the order of seconds), and perhaps a much wider network deals with demands on memory involving longer time frames. In a footnote in our preceding chapter, we described the distributed connectivity found when Selemon and Goldman-Rakic (1988) studied prefrontal and parietal lobes in anterograde fashion. A perspective from thalamus is interesting in such demonstrations of distributed networks, because of a consistency: whether information *heads to* cortex (Goldman-Rakic and Porrino, 1985) or *from* cortex (Selemon and Goldman-Rakic,

---

[22] Not discussed previously is a provocative claim (Von Neumann's) about the breadth and depth of biological memory. There's evidence, he says (he doesn't present the evidence, yet the following statement rings true somehow), "that there is *no true forgetting in the nervous system* . . . impressions once received may be removed from . . . the center of attention, *but not truly erased . . .*" (my emphasis, Von Neumann, 2000, p. 63). He audaciously estimated that memory in the course of sixty years of life totaled 2.8×10^{20} bits.

The verifiable reliability of memory is another matter.

1988), higher order nuclei of thalamus are involved. As Jules Luys illustrated in the 19th century, thalamus is central like a pivot, both anatomically and operationally. Such has been Sherman and Guillery's career-long point of view, as we have tried to summarize.

*

Goldman-Rakic and Porrino (1985) were interested that some thalamic nuclei distinguish themselves from others because of their growth and differentiation across species:

> A role for the mediodorsal (MD) nucleus of the thalamus in the cognitive and emotional life of the individual was suggested nearly a century ago and is increasingly supported by contemporary evidence of the MD's specific participation in the memory systems of the human brain. In keeping with both its affective and cognitive functions, the mediodorsal nucleus reaches its peak dimensions and cytoarchitectonic complexity in the human brain in parallel with the expansion of the prefrontal cortex to which it projects.

In a rudimentary way, it *is* possible to distinguish nuclei that have undergone phylogenetic growth disproportionately in primates and humans—a short list includes medial dorsal nucleus, *centre médian* nucleus, and pulvinar. Goldman-Rakic and Porrino refer to cases in which memory-related or associational, as opposed to comparatively elementary (first-order?) thalamic nuclei, degenerate in progressive thalamic dementias.

*

We can learn much about the implications of prefrontal expansion by turning to an early, single example of such a disease process (Stern, 1939).

A 41 year-old man presented to hospital in February, 1938. He had been healthy and energetic, without family history of neurological or other disease. He had worked in a chemist's shop, perhaps helping to dispense prescriptions.

In May of the preceding year, he described a feeling of "being run down" and "in need of rest." By July, he was "more inert . . . always licking his lips and complaining of his mouth being dry." Thirst and polyuria followed for the next two months, during which time he became increasingly drowsy. By August, he gave up work, then spoke less and less, but he filled enlarging gaps in his memory with confabulations. He became unable to write and couldn't read.

There's a transcript of an interaction with him at the time of admission:

Q: What is your name? A: (Answered correctly.)
Q: How old are you? A: "Eighteen." (Ten minutes later said "eight or nine.")
Q: Where are you? A: "Just thinking where I'd like to be."
Q: How long have you been here ? A: "Four or six months."
Q: Where were you before? A: "The room very similar to the other one, but perhaps a different build."
. . .
Q: What is the date? A: "Jan. 25 or 26, I think."
Q: What year? A: "203." (Persists in 203 to repeated questioning.)
Q: Who is the King? A: "King George."
Q: What number? A: "209." [The British king in 1938 was George VI.]
Q: When did the War begin? A: "209."
Q: How long did it last? A: "209."
Q: When did it finish? A: "About 209—I can't think about that like I do about other things."

Throughout the interview, he appeared restless, continually adjusted bedsheets, or he rubbed his head and face. He exhibited sucking motions of the mouth and "grotesque" arm and hand gestures. He stuck out his tongue when asked, but then stuck out his tongue "for some time" in response to other requests.

His elementary neurological examination was notable for mid-sized pupils that didn't react to light or accommodation. His extraocular movements were full. Power was normal. He often "introduced perverse movements." Rooting and grasp reflexes were present. Deep tendon reflexes were brisk, especially in the arms. Plantar responses were colored by voluntary posturing and withdrawal. He wasn't ataxic. Sensation "could not be tested."

The examination didn't much change until he lapsed into coma, then died.

*

Respectfully, one could speak of a clinico-pathological de-correlation in this case. There was no evidence of pretectal or cranial nuclear abnormality to explain the iridoplegia both to light and accommodation. For all the frontal-release phenomena observed, though cortex and subcortical white matter weren't uninvolved, the striking pathological aspect was almost complete neuronal loss of many, but not all thalamic nuclei bilaterally. Anterior, medial dorsal, *centre médian*, lateral nuclei, posterior nuclear group, and pulvinar as well, all based on Stern's camera lucida drawings in figure 2 and figures 1 and 3-5) had "disappeared," replaced by gliosis. Ventral tier nuclei (presumably VA, VL, and VP) and MGN and LGN were preserved, as was the reticular nucleus.

A progressive dementia with frontal features (and sleepiness, then coma) involves thalamic connections to phylogenetically newer cortex. Stern's conclusion borrows from Le Gros Clark (1932), who ended a famous monograph in *Brain* with a treatment of medial dorsal nucleus and prefrontal lobe. He opined that there can't be any thalamic nuclear homolog to medial dorsal nucleus in a submammalian brain, simply because a prefrontal cortex appears too late in phylogeny.

In evolutionary terms, newer categories or anatomies of processing emerge in the phylogenetically recent human thalamocortex.[23]

---

[23]   In ontogeny as well, particularly in the development of cortical resting states observed in functional images, preterm intracortical activity is minimal in contrast to adults, whose resting states are driven less by peripheral input than by recurrent interactions of thalamus and cortex (Colonese and Khazipov, 2012).

Appendix

Semiology of an Acute Thalamic Lesion

What clinical signs might be expected from a lesion such as this?

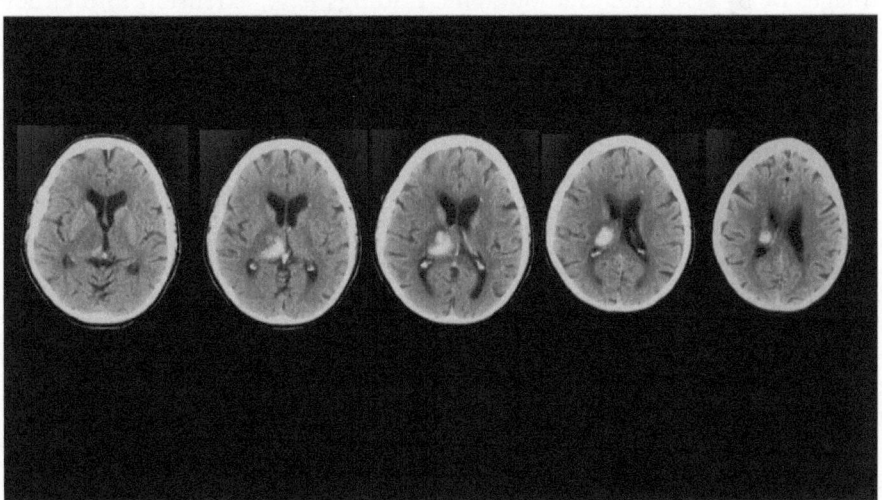

Osawa and Maeshima (2016) reported 115 cases of thalamic hemorrhages, studied only with CT imaging (cases accrued from 2008 to 2012); 44 had right thalamic hemorrhages. Of those 44, four had blood in right thalamus; in 36, blood extended into internal capsule; and four cases showed extension into midbrain. In just over half (54%), blood had ruptured into the lateral ventricle. The authors observed that 35 of their 44 (79%) exhibited neglect, as evaluated by a Behavioural Inattention Test (Wilson et al., 1987) administered soon after presentation, within a day in most cases. Nine right thalamic hemorrhages did not exhibit neglect.

Reviewing their experience against earlier reports, the same authors (Maeshima and Osawa, 2018) cite Kumral et al. (1995), who observed neglect of various types in roughly a third of 51 right-sided lesions in a series of 100 consecutive cases of acute thalamic hemorrhage. Clinical assessment included double simultaneous stimulation (auditory, tactile, and visual), a line bisection task, and determination of gnosis of the left hemibody. Of the 51, ten were anosognosic for contralateral hemiparesis; 17 neglected contralateral visual hemispace and were also judged to be anosognosic; only two had visuospatial neglect exclusively. Tactile and visual extinction were noted in 14; extinction to auditory stimuli happened in ten. In total, 19 of 51 demonstrated some type of neglect syndrome.

As has been observed by several groups (Osawa and Maeshima, 2016; Chung et al., 1996; Kawahara et al. 1986, Walshe et al., 1977), hemorrhage size relates to presentation. Whether judged by actual measurements on images or by associated radiographic findings (e.g., extension into either internal capsule, ventricle, or both), larger lesions were associated with the clearest clinical deficits, whether motor or sensory signs or neglect (the last specifically in right thalamic lesions). In terms of smaller lesions, Kawahara et al.'s (1986) case 4 is illustrative:

> A 61 year-old, right-handed man with a history of untreated hypertension presented with nausea, headache, and a minimal left hemiparesis (the last resolved within hours). He was awake, alert, and fluent in speech; eye movements were normal; there was no sensory loss with double simultaneous stimulation. "The next day, he walked to the toilet; he got lost on the way back to his room, even though he said he know the way back (topographic memory disturbance)." Copying pictures on a page was difficult for him; no dressing disorder, ideomotor apraxia, unilateral spatial neglect, or agnosia (tactile, color, or object) was noted. CT found a hemorrhage in right dorsal thalamus involving lateral posterior and dorsomedial nuclei as well as the pulvinar.

*

Lesion location within thalamus is different consideration. Tokgoz et al. (2013) retrospectively studied 101 cases of thalamic hemorrhage from 1992-2012 (56 on the right) to find that medial bleeds or those globally involving a thalamus were most often associated with extension into a ventricle, but the authors did not provide detailed clinical correlations for their cohort of right hemorrhages. In Chung et al.'s series (1996) of 175 patients, 14% had paramedian (right or left) bleeds, many with extension of blood into the third ventricle or into midbrain. Forty-four per cent had posterolateral (right or left) hematomas, often with rupture into the posterior horn of lateral ventricle and extension into the posterior limb of internal capsule. In those cases, fatality rates were high (35%); sensory and motor signs in the contralateral hemibody were "marked," hemineglect was observed with right hematomas (in 20 of 35 cases, 57%) and a language problem with left hematomas (in 18 of 42 cases, 43%). Hirose et al. (1985) reported six cases of posterior thalamic hemorrhage associated with relatively benign clinical outcome in five; all patients exhibited sensory deficits contralateral to the lesion, gaze preference toward the side of the lesion, hypometric saccades away from the side of the lesion, and reduced optokinetic nystagmus towards the side of the lesion. The authors glossed the ophthalmological findings as interruption of fibers descending in the vicinity of posterior thalamus from frontal eye fields and parietooccipital cortex. Horner's syndrome on the same side of the lesion manifested in four the six, and was attributed to compressive effects on ipsilateral hypothalamus.

Posterolateral thalamic hemorrhages can disturb the subjective perception of verticality of posture. First described in the stroke rehabilitation literature, a minority of hemiparetic patients had been observed to push themselves with a nonparetic arm towards the paretic side, for example, when seated. Even when standing, "pushers" resisted others' attempts to correct their tilted axial posture–the tilt typically 20 degrees towards the side of the lesion, away from both the midline with respect to gravity and away from the hemiparetic side. Change in the subjective perception of the visual vertical had been described previously in stroke, vestibular disease, and migraine, but contraversive pushing (towards the side of paresis) led to a thought of a separate graviceptive system in humans (Karnath et al., 2000). The percept of the visual vertical can be preserved when that of the postural vertical is skewed, as the percept of the postural vertical can be retained when that of the visual vertical is amiss.

Over a three-year period, Karnath et al. (2005) then prospectively evaluated 40 consecutive thalamic strokes. Fourteen patients "pushed" (the majority with large, posterior thalamic hemorrhages; only two with ischemic infarcts); 26 did not (in the latter group, 20 had infarcts). Many, not all, cases of right thalamic stroke (infarction and hemorrhage) exhibited contralateral spatial neglect (9 of 23); some, not all, cases of left thalamic stroke had unspecified aphasias (6 of 17).

Literature regarding the presentation of ischemic infarction as opposed to hemorrhage (bland infarcts of course can convert to hemorrhagic ones) has its own rich past of descriptions. Dating to the very early 20th century, Dejerine and Roussy, along with Foix and Hillemand a few years later, described a thalamic syndrome resulting from infarction with *many* aspects, as summarized by Amici (2012): abnormal movements (chorea, dystonia, athetosis, tremor, myoclonus), limb "oscillations" (and other adventitious movements, sometimes presenting weeks to months after stroke per Kim, 2001), mixed sensorimotor deficits with or without pain, hemiataxia, hypermetria, dysdiadochokinesis, disturbances in station and gait ("thalamic astasia"), even *la main thalamique*, a hand that is flexed and pronated with the thumb buried beneath flexed fingers, all in addition to a spectral array of levels of disturbed consciousness and a variety of internal and external oculomotor abnormalities as well as sometimes incomplete visual field deficits, including "sectoranopsias."

In the current century, groups have attempted to characterize the behavioral (Carrera and Bogousslavsky, 2006) and higher cognitive (Karussis et al., 2000; Amici et al., 2003) deficits associated with thalamic infarction, with mixed success. Whether observed disturbances are indeed aphasic, visuospatial, or the result of an impaired "realization of codes" due to susceptibility to "the immediate influence of outside stimuli and former traces" (Luria, 1977) remains an open question. Based on a review of 60 cases dating to 1980 selected because of specific and rigorous neuropsychological as opposed to simpler bedside assessments, Van der Werf et al. (2000), opined that executive *frontal* dysfunction correlated with medial dorsal or intralaminar nuclear injury, contrary the traditional notion that those nuclei are non-specific in their projections. Groenewegen and Berendse (1994) have likewise argued that midline and intralaminar thalamic nuclei are quite specific in their connections with limbic/ventral *corpus striatum* and prefrontal cortex.

In thalamic lesions, expectation of a clinical sign (neglect in a right lesion, a language disturbance in a left lesion) is partially, but not wholly supported by retrospective and prospective series. If a right lesion *can* result or *often* results in neglect, why should there be cases in which no neglect is evident, even if strokes are of similar size and location? DeWitte et al. (2010) applied exclusions to a database of 465 reports of thalamic stroke dating to 1980; perhaps the most rigorous of their criteria was a requirement that neuropsychological evaluation using specific testing batteries be delayed to no shorter than three weeks after and no longer than four months after stroke.[24] Of the 465, only 42 qualified for further analysis; nearly all were left thalamic strokes with only five non-left cases (two involving right thalamus, three were bilateral). Aside from aspects of a language disturbance (dysnomia in 72.2%, problems with writing in 65%, and with comprehension in 43.8%), the authors also observed that 44% of the left cases exhibited features more typically associated with a non-dominant hemispheric disorder (visual neglect and disturbances in visual memory) and 64.3% exhibited a constructional apraxia.

Given such observations, in concert with the known, protean manifestations of thalamic pathology, is there any paradigm regarding semiology to aid our localization?

Though support for the idea is preliminary, it may be that a clinician needs more useful information, not about the lesion, but about the brain as a whole in the context of an acute change. In a report related to aphasia or neglect after thalamic stroke (Sebastian et al., 2014), neglect only in two (of ten) cases of right thalamic infarction was associated with cortical hypoperfusion in diffusion-weighted and perfusion-weighted imaging obtained simultaneously within 24 hours of presentation. Among five (of ten) cases of *left* thalamic infarction, only one case exhibited an associated cortical perfusion deficit.

---

[24] The authors' rational had to do with excluding hyperacute or acute effects, such as diaschisis, a phenomenon in which neurophysiological effects manifest at a distance from a focal lesion. The concept of diaschisis has been reviewed in depth (Carrera and Tononi, 2014); it could account not only for unexpected clinical semiology at presentation, but also may predict for longer-term outcomes–e.g., less hypometabolic diaschisis, better prognosis.

*

The patient whose CT begins this chapter had no abnormalities on elementary neurological examination, including an assessment of extinction to double simultaneous stimulation (visually and to touch). There was no disturbance in attention, language, constructional or dressing praxis, strength, coordination, station, or gait. Her only complaint, aside from headache, was that she could not ascertain how to lie down in bed. When asked to demonstrate her problem, she approached a hospital bed perpendicular to its long axis, then positioned herself on all fours on the bed surface. When asked what she planned to do next, she said, "I don't have any idea."

The axial section furthest to the left in the image corresponds either to Talairach and Tournoux figure 118 or 119 (Talairach and Tournoux, 1988). Territory supplied by thalamoperforate (paramedian) arteries appears spared, including ventral nuclei such as **VA**, **VL**, and **VP** as well as part of **MD** and intralaminar nuclei (e.g., **CeM**) at this level. More dorsally, various nuclei are obscured by blood, including **A**, **LD**, dorsal **MD**, perhaps dorsal parts of **VA**, **VL**, **VP**, and **Plm**, **Pll**, and **Po**.

*

She does enter the bed. On all fours, she does not lie down.

Students of language will note the change to present tense in the italicized summary and the use of *anaphora*, the repetition of "*she does*" along with the recognition that "she" in both sentences refers to the same person. Psychological research (e.g., Kelter et al., 2004) has explored memory dynamics in descriptions of unfolding occurrences: a protagonist's current situation (that described in the second sentence) proves more accessible than other (anaphoric) antecedents in time or space. In the event of a boundary between events—perhaps just entering bed—, retrieval of prior information may be compromised in the way that walking through a door can dim recall about the reason for entering (Thompson and Radvansky, 2016; Pettijohn and Radvansky, 2018). Location-updating effects occur in normal persons, and can manifest as a forme fruste of memory disturbance. Subjective boundaries become inconsistent and idiosyncratic in aging and in dementia (Radvansky and Zachs, 2017).

Once in bed, she does not unfold from all fours. Zachs and Tversky (2001) offer this view:

> The world presents nothing but continuity and flux, yet we seem to perceive activity as consisting of discrete events that have some orderly relations. This ability guides our understanding of what is happening, helps control our actions in the midst of it, and forms the basis of our later recollection of what took place. An inability to perceive events as such would be even more debilitating than an inability to perceive . . .[.]

But is it abnormal, too, that she gets in bed on all fours as opposed to sitting at its edge? What is the beginning of ordered relations involved in simply lying down? Does her problem relate to the perception of herself in space, her knowledge of what to do in a sequence, or both together? If the last, then we might visualize a lesion at the highly trafficked interface between perception and action.

References

Images

\<Image 1 page 15.\> The anatomical image is adapted from http://brains. anatomy.msu.edu/brains/human/coronal/2240_cell.html, and is used with permission from The Human Brain Atlas, part of the brain collections of the National Museum of Health and Medicine, Michigan State University, and the University of Wisconsin. These collections are available online at http://brainmuseum.org, http://brains.rad.msu.edu, and/or http:// neurosciencelibrary.org, and are supported by the National Science Foundation and the National Institutes of Health.

\<Image 4 page 29.\> The image is adapted from https://wellcomecollection. org/works/cgnp3kxm/items?canvas=119&langCode=ger&sierraId= b21461296[.] Public domain.

\<Image 5 page 38.\> The anatomical image is adapted from http:// neurosciencelibrary.org//Specimens/PRIMATES/RHESUSMonkey/ brain/Rhesusmonk6.jpg, and is used with permission from The Human Brain Atlas, part of the brain collections of the National Museum of Health and Medicine, Michigan State University, and the University of Wisconsin. These collections are available online at http://brainmuseum. org, http://brains.rad.msu.edu, and/or http://neurosciencelibrary.org, and are supported by the National Science Foundation and the National Institutes of Health.

\<Image 6 page 42.\> The anatomical image is adapted from

http://brains.anatomy.msu.edu/brains/human/coronal/1840_fiber.html, and is used with permission from The Human Brain Atlas, part of the brain collections of the National Museum of Health and Medicine, Michigan State University, and the University of Wisconsin. These collections are available online at http://brainmuseum.org, http://brains.rad.msu.edu, and/or http://neurosciencelibrary.org, and are supported by the National Science Foundation and the National Institutes of Health.

<Image 7 page 44.> The anatomical image is adapted from

http://brains.anatomy.msu.edu/brains/human/coronal/2000_fiber.html, and is used with permission from The Human Brain Atlas, part of the brain collections of the National Museum of Health and Medicine, Michigan State University, and the University of Wisconsin. These collections are available online at http://brainmuseum.org, http://brains.rad.msu.edu, and/or http://neurosciencelibrary.org, and are supported by the National Science Foundation and the National Institutes of Health.

<Image 8 page 47.> The anatomical image is adapted from

http://brains.anatomy.msu.edu/brains/human/coronal/2060_fiber.html, and is used with permission from The Human Brain Atlas, part of the brain collections of the National Museum of Health and Medicine, Michigan State University, and the University of Wisconsin. These collections are available online at http://brainmuseum.org, http://brains.rad.msu.edu, and/or http://neurosciencelibrary.org, and are supported by the National Science Foundation and the National Institutes of Health.

<Image 9 page 49.> The anatomical image is adapted from

http://brains.anatomy.msu.edu/brains/human/coronal/2240_fiber.html, and is used with permission from The Human Brain Atlas, part of the brain collections of the National Museum of Health and Medicine, Michigan State University, and the University of Wisconsin. These collections are available online at http://brainmuseum.org, http://brains.rad.msu.edu, and/or http://neurosciencelibrary.org, and are supported by the National Science Foundation and the National Institutes of Health.

<Image 10 page 50.> The image is adapted from https://wellcomecollection.org/works/aymhzmcz/items?canvas=41&langCode=fre&sierraId=b21214098 [.] Public domain.

<Image 11 page 53.> The image is adapted from http://brains.anatomy.msu.edu/brains/human/coronal/2390_fiber.html, and is used with permission from The Human Brain Atlas, part of the brain collections of the National Museum of Health and Medicine, Michigan State University, and the University of Wisconsin. These collections are available online at http://brainmuseum.org, http://brains.rad.msu.edu, and/or http://neurosciencelibrary.org, and are supported by the National Science Foundation and the National Institutes of Health.

<Image 14 page 62.> The image to the left is adapted from

http://neurosciencelibrary.org//specimens/primates/owlmonkey/sections/101_OWLMONK_69-255.JPG and the image to the right is adapted from

http://neurosciencelibrary.org//specimens/primates/owlmonkey/sections/500_OWLMONK_69-255.JPG, and is used with permission from The Human Brain Atlas, part of the brain collections of the National Museum of Health and Medicine, Michigan State University, and the University of Wisconsin. These collections are available online at http://brainmuseum.org, http://brains.rad.msu.edu, and/or http://neurosciencelibrary.org, and are supported by the National Science Foundation and the National Institutes of Health.

<Image 15-18 page 63-64.> The anatomical image to the left in each is adapted from

http://neurosciencelibrary.org//specimens/primates/owlmonkey/sections/101_OWLMONK_69-255.JPG, and is used with permission from The Human Brain Atlas, part of the brain collections of the National Museum of Health and Medicine, Michigan State University, and the University of Wisconsin. These collections are available online at http://brainmuseum.org, http://brains.rad.msu.edu, and/or http://

neurosciencelibrary.org, and are supported by the National Science Foundation and the National Institutes of Health.

Books and Monographs

Carpenter, Malcolm B. and Sutin, Jerome. *Human Neuroanatomy*. [8th ed.] Baltimore and London: Williams and Wilkins, 1983.

Ebenstein, Alan. *Hayek's Journey. The Mind of Friedrich Hayek*. New York: Palgrave Macmillan, 2003.

Flechsig, Paul. *Gehirn und Seele*. Leipzig: Verlag von Veit and Comp., 1896.

Hayek, F[riedrich]. A[ugust]. *The Sensory Order. An Inquiry into the Foundations of Theoretical Psychology*. Chicago: University of Chicago Press, 1976.

Hayek, F.A. *New Studies in Philosophy, Politics, Economics and the History of Ideas*. London, Melbourne and Henley: Routledge and Kegan Paul, 1978.

Hayek, F.A. *Hayek on Hayek. An Autobiographical Dialogue*. [Eds. Stephen Kresge and Leif Wenar.] Chicago and London: University of Chicago Press, 1994.

Haymaker, Webb [ed.]. *The Founders of Neurology. One Hundred and Thirty-Three Biographical Sketches*. Springfield: Charles C. Thomas, 1953.

Helmholtz, H[ermann von]. *Popular Lectures on Scientific Subjects* [2nd ed.]. Trans. E. Atkinson. London: Longmans, Green, and Co., 1881.

Jones, Edward G. *The Thalamus* [Volumes I and II]. New York: SpringerScience+Business Media, 1985 [facsimile edition of original publication by Plenum Press, New York, also in 1985].

Luys, Jules Bernard. *Le Cerveau et Ses Fonctions* [5th *éd.*]. Paris: G. Bailliere, 1882 [English translation: Luys, Jules Bernard. *The Brain and Its Functions*. New York: D. Appleton, 1882].

Mach, Ernst. *The Analysis of Sensations and the Relation of the Physical to the Psychical*. Trans. C.M. Williams [from the first German edition; revised and supplemented from the fifth German edition by S. Waterlow]. Chicago and London: Open Court, 1914, reprinted by Forgotten Books (no city of publication), 2012.

Marey, E[tienne] J[ules]. *La Méthode graphique dans les sciences expérimentales et principalement en physiologie et en médicine*. Paris: G. Masson, 1885. (Pages specifically cited in the text refer to a subchapter entitled *"Applications. –Graphique du mouvement des trains sur les chemins de fer."*)

Morowitz, Harold J. and Singer, Jerome L. [eds.] *The Mind, the Brain, and Complex Adaptive Systems* [Proceedings Volume XXII Santa Fe Institute Studies in the Sciences of Complexity]. Reading: Addison-Wesley, 1995.

Nieuwenhuys, Rudolf, Voogd, Jan, and van Huijzen, Christiaan. *The Human Central Nervous System*. Fourth ed. Berlin/Heidelberg/New York: Springer Verlag, 2008.

Nolte, John. *The Human Brain. An Introduction to Its Functional Anatomy*. [4th ed.] St. Louis: Mosby, 1999.

Schaltenbrand, Georges and Wahren, Waldemar (with the cooperation of L.V. Amador and I.A. Blundell). *Atlas for Stereotaxy of the Human Brain* [2nd ed., revised and enlarged]. Stuttgart: Georg Thieme, 1977.

Schaltenbrand, Georges and Wahren, Waldemar (with the cooperation of L.V. Amador and I.A. Blundell). *Guide to the Atlas for Stereotaxy of the Human Brain* [2nd ed., revised and enlarged]. Stuttgart: Georg Thieme, 1977a.

Shepherd, Gordon M. [ed.]. *The Synaptic Organization of the Brain* [4th ed.]. New York and Oxford: Oxford University Press, 1998.

Sherman, S. Murray and Guillery, R[ainer].W[alter]. *Exploring the Thalamus and Its Role in Cortical Function* [2nd ed.]. Cambridge and London: MIT Press, 2006.

———

Sherman, S. Murray and Guillery, R[ainer].W[alter]. *Functional Connections of Cortical Areas. A New View from the Thalamus*. Cambridge and London: MIT Press, 2013.

Sporns, Olaf. *Networks of the Brain*. Cambridge and London: MIT Press, 2011.

Talairach, Jean and Tournoux, Pierre. *Co-Planar Stereotaxic Atlas of the Human Brain. 3-Dimensional Proportional System: An Approach to Cerebral Imaging*. Trans. Mark Rayport. Stuttgart and New York: Georg Thieme Verlag, 1988.

Von Neumann, John. *The Computer and the Brain* [2nd ed.]. New Haven and London: Yale Nota Bene/Yale University Press, 2000 [original publication in 1958].

Wilson B, Cockburn J, Halligan P. *Behavioral Inattention Test*. London: Thames Valley Test Company, 1987.

Articles and Chapters in Books

Abivardi A and Bach DR. Deconstructing white matter connectivity of human amygdala nuclei with thalamus and cortex subdivisions in vivo. *Human Brain Mapping* 2017;38:3927-3940.

Alcaraz F, Marchand AR, Courtand G, Coutureau E, Wolff M. Parallel inputs from the mediodorsal thalamus to the prefrontal cortex in the rat. *European Journal of Neuroscience* 2016;44:1972-1986.

Amici S. Thalamic infarcts and hemorrhages. *Frontiers of Neurology and Neuroscience* 2012;30:132-136.

Annoni J-M, Khateb A, Gramigna S, Staub F, Carota A, Maeder P, Bogousslavsky J. Chronic cognitive impairment following laterothalamic infarcts. *Archives of Neurology* 2003;60:1439-1443.

Birner J. The surprising place of cognitive psychology in the work of F.A. Hayek. *History of Economic Ideas* 1999;7:43-84.

Bogousslavsky J, Regli F, Uske A. Thalamic infarcts: clinical syndromes, etiology, and prognosis. *Neurology* 1988;38:837-848.

Carrera E and Bogousslavsky J. The thalamus and behavior. Effects of anatomically distinct strokes. *Neurology* 2006;66:1817-1823.

Carrera E and Tononi G. Diaschisis: past, present, future. *Brain* 2014;137:2408-2422.

Castaigne P, Lhermitte F, Buge A, Escourolle R, Hauw JJ, Lyon-Caen O. Paramedian thalamic and midbrain infarcts: clinical and neuropathological study. *Annals of Neurology* 1981;10:127-148.

Çavdar S, Özgür M, Uysal SP, Amuk ÖG. Motor afferents from the cerebellum, zona incerta and substantia nigra to the mediodorsal thalamic nucleus in the rat. *Journal of Integrative Neuroscience* 2014;13:565-578.

Chung C-S, Caplan LR, Han W, Pessin MS, Lee K-H, Kim J-M. Thalamic haemorrhage. *Brain* 1996;119:1873-1886.

Colonnese M and Khazipov R. Spontaneous activity in developing sensory circuits: implications for resting state fMRI. *Neuroimage* 2012;62:2212-2221.

DeWitte L, Brouns R, Kavadis D, Engelborghs S, DeDeyn P, Mariën P. Cognitive, affective and behavioural disturbances following vascular thalamic lesions: a review. *Cortex* 2011;47:273-319.

Douard JW. E.-J. Marey's visual rhetoric and the graphic decomposition of the body. *Studies in the History of the Philosophy of Science* 1995;26:175-204.

Ebenstein A. Epistemology, psychology, and methodology. In: *Hayek's Journey. The Mind of Friedrich Hayek*. New York: Palgrave Macmillan, 2003, pp. 127-138.

Faull RLM and Mehler WR. The cells of origin of nigrotectal, nigrothalamic, and nigrostriatal projections in the rat. *Neuroscience* 1978;3:989-1002.

Funahashi S. Prefrontal contribution to decision-making under free-choice conditions. *Frontiers in Neuroscience* 26 July 2017, https://doi.org/10.3389/fnins2017.00431[.]

Funahashi S, Bruce CJ, Goldman-Rakic PS. Mnemonic coding of visual space in the monkey's dorsolateral prefrontal cortex. *Journal of Neurophysiology* 1989;61:331-348.

Funahashi S, Bruce CJ, Goldman-Rakic PS. Dorsolateral prefrontal lesions and oculomotor delayed-response performance: evidence for mnemonic "scotomas." *Journal of Neuroscience* 1993;13:1479-1497.

Funahashi S, Chafee MV, Goldman-Rakic PS. Prefrontal neuronal activity in rhesus monkeys performing a delayed anti-saccade task. *Nature* 1993a;365(6448):753-756.

Goldman-Rakic PS. Neurobiology of mental representation. In: *The Mind, the Brain, and Complex Adaptive Systems* [Proceedings Volume XXII Santa Fe Institute Studies in the Sciences of Complexity]. Reading: Addison-Wesley, 1995, pp. 51-62.

Goldman-Rakic P. The "psychic cell" of Ramón y Cajal. *Progress in Brain Research* 2002;136:427-434.

Goldman-Rakic PS, Funahashi S, Bruce CJ. Neocortical memory circuits. *Cold Spring Harbor Symposia on Quantitative Biology* 1990;55:1025-1038.

Goldman-Rakic PS and Porrino LJ. The primate mediodorsal (MD) nucleus and its projection to the frontal lobe. *Journal of Comparative Neurology* 1985;242:535-560.

Groenewegen HJ and Berendse HW. The specificity of the 'nonspecific' midline and intralaminar thalamic nuclei. *Trends in Neurosciences* 1994;17:52-57.

Guillery RW. Patterns of fiber degeneration in the dorsal lateral geniculate nucleus of the cat following lesions in the visual cortex. *Journal of Comparative Neurology* 1967;130:197-221.

Guillery R.W. Anatomical pathways that link perception and action. *Progress in Brain Research* 2005;149:235-256.

Guo K, Yamawaki N, Svoboda K, Shepherd GMG. Anterolateral motor cortex connects with a medial subdivision of ventromedial thalamus through cell type-specific circuits, forming an excitatory thalamo-cortico-thalamic loop via layer 1 apical tuft dendrites of layer 5B pyramidal tract type neurons. *Journal of Neuroscience* 2018;38:8787-8797.

Hayek FA. An outline of the theory. In: *The Sensory Order. An Inquiry into the Foundations of Theoretical Psychology.* Chicago: University of Chicago Press, 1976a, pp. 37-54.

Hayek FA. The nervous system as an instrument of classification. In: *The Sensory Order. An Inquiry into the Foundations of Theoretical Psychology.* Chicago: University of Chicago Press, 1976b, pp. 55-78.

Hayek, F.A. The primacy of the abstract. In: *New Studies in Philosophy, Politics, Economics and the History of Ideas.* London, Melbourne and Henley: Routledge and Kegan Paul, 1978, pp. 35-49.

Heredia R, Real MÁ, Suárez J, Guirado S, Dávila JC. A proposed homology between the reptilian dorsomedial thalamic nucleus and the mammalian paraventricular nucleus. *Brain Research Bulletin* 2002;57:443-445.

Hikosaka O. The habenula: from stress evasion to value-based decision-making. *Nature Reviews Neuroscience* 2010;11:503-513.

Hirose G, Kosoegawa H, Saeki M, Kitagawa Y, Oda R, Kanda S, Matsuhira T. The syndrome of posterior thalamic hemorrhage. *Neurology* 1985;35:998-1002.

Hsu DT and Price JL. Paraventricular thalamic nucleus: subcortical connections and innervation by serotonin, orexin, and corticotropin releasing hormone in Macaque monkeys. *Journal of Comparative /Neurology* 2009;512:825-848.

Hu F, Kamigaki T, Zhang Z, Zhang S, Dan U, Dan Y. Prefrontal corticotectal neurons enhance visual processing through the superior colliculus and pulvinar thalamus. *Neuron* 2019;104:1141-1152.

Hunnicutt BJ, Long BR, Kusefoglu D, Gertz KJ, Zhong H, Mao T. A comprehensive thalamocortical projection map at the mesoscopic level. *Nature Neuroscience* 2014;17:1276-1285.

Impieri D, Gamberini M, Passarelli L, Rosa MGP, Galletti C. Thalamo-cortical projections to the macaque superior parietal lobule areas PEc and PE. *Journal of Comparative Neurology* 2018;526:1041-1056.

Jacobsen CF. Studies of cerebral function in primates. *Comparative Psychology Monographs* 1936;13:1-68.

Jankowski MM, Passecker J, Islam MN, Vann S, Erichsen JT, Aggleton JP, O'Mara SM. Evidence for spatially-responsive neurons in the rostral thalamus. *Frontiers in Behavioral Neuroscience* 13 October 2015, doi: 10.3389/fnbeh.2015.00256[.]

Jones EG. Lateral geniculate nucleus. In: *The Thalamus* [Volume II]. New York: SpringerScience+Business Media, 1985a, pp. 453-527.

Jones EG. Principles of thalamic organization. In: *The Thalamus* [Volume I]. New York: SpringerScience+Business Media, 1985b, pp. 85-149.

Karnath H-O, Ferber S, Dichgans J. The origin of contraversive pushing. Evidence for a second graviceptive system in humans. *Neurology* 2000;55:1298-1304.

Karnath H-O, Johannsen L, Broetz D, Küker W. Posterior thalamic hemorrhage induces "pusher syndrome." *Neurology* 2005;64:1014-1019.

Karussis D, Leker RR, Abramsky O. Cognitive dysfunction following thalamic stroke: a study of 16 cases and review of the literature. *Journal of the Neurological Sciences* 2000;172:25-29.

Kass JH and Baldwin MKL. The evolution of the pulvinar complex in primates and its role in the dorsal and ventral streams of cortical processing. *Vision* 2020;4; doi:10.3390/vision4010003[.]

Kawahara N, Sato K, Muraki M, Tanaka K, Kaneko M, Uemura K. CT classification of small thalamic hemorrhages and their clinical implications. *Neurology* 1986;36:165-172.

Kim JS. Delayed onset mixed mixed involuntary movements after thalamic stroke: clinical, radiological and pathophysiological findings. *Brain* 2001;124:299-309.

Krieg WJS. Jules Bernard Luys (1828-1897). In: *The Founders of Neurology. One Hundred and Thirty-Three Biographical Sketches*. Springfield: Charles C. Thomas, 1953, pp. 55-58.

Kumral E, Kocaer T, Ertübey NÖ, Kumral K. Thalamic hemorrhage. A prospective study of 100 patients. *Stroke* 1995;26:964-970.

Kuramoto E, Pan S, Furuta T, Tanaka YR, Iwai H, Yamanaka A, Ohno S, Kaneko T, Goto T, Hioki H. Individual mediodorsal thalamic neurons project to multiple areas of the rat prefrontal cortex: a single neuron-tracing study using virus vectors. *Journal of Comparative Neurology* 2017;525:166-185.

Lakatos P, O'Connell MN, Barczak A. Pondering the pulvinar. *Neuron* 2016;89:5-7.

Lee J, Wang W, Sabatini BL. Anatomically segregated basal ganglia pathways allow parallel behavioral modulation. *Nature Neuroscience* 2020, Sep 28. doi: 10.1038/s41593-020-00712-5.

Le Gros Clark WE. The structure and connections of the thalamus. *Brain* 1932;55:406-470.

Luria AR. On quasi-aphasic speech disturbances in lesions of the deep structures of the brain. *Brain and Language* 1977;4:432-459.

Maeshima S and Osawa A. Thalamic lesions and aphasia or neglect. *Current Neurology and Neuroscience Reports* 2018;18:39 [on-line publication].

Mandelbaum G, Teranda J, Haynes TM, Hochbaum DR, Huang KW, Hyun M, Venkataraju KU, Straub C, Wang W, Robertson K, Osten P, Sabatini BL. Distinct cortical-thalamic-striatal circuits through the parafascicular nucleus. *Neuron* 2019;102:636-652.

Mayer A, Lewenfus G, Bittencourt-Navarrete RE, Clasca F, Franca JGD. Thalamic inputs to posterior parietal cortical areas involved in skilled forelimb movement and tool use in the Capuchin monkey. *Cerebral Cortex* 2019;29:5098-5115.

Mo C and Sherman SM. A sensorimotor pathway via higher-order thalamus. *Journal of Neuroscience* 2019;39:692-704.

Monavarfeshani A, Sabbagh U, Fox MA. Not a one-trick pony: diverse connectivity and functions of the lateral geniculate complex. *Visual Neuroscience* 2017;34:E012, doi:10.1017/S0952523817000098[.]

Nakajima M and Halassa MM. Thalamic control of functional cortical connectivity. *Current Opinion in Neurobiology* 2017;44:127-131.

Nakamura H. Cerebellar projections to the ventral lateral geniculate nucleus and the thalamic reticular nucleus in the cat. *Journal of Neuroscience Research* 2018;96:63-74.

Nacimento ES, Duarte RB, Silva SF, Engelberth RCGJ, Toledo CAB, Calvacante JS, Costa MSMO. Retinal projections to the thalamic paraventricular nucleus in the rock cavy (*Kerodon rupestris*). *Brain Research* 2008;1241:56-61.

Ogundele OM, Lee CC, Francis J. Thalamic dopaminergic neurons projects [sic] to the paraventricular nucleus-rostral ventrolateral medulla/C1 neural circuit. *The Anatomical Record* 2017;300:1307-1314.

O'Mara SM and Aggleton JP. Space and memory (far) beyond the hippocampus: many subcortical structures also support cognitive mapping and mnemonic processing. *Frontiers in Neural Circuits* 07 August 2019, https://doi.org/10.3389/fncir.2019.00052[.]

Osawa A and Maeshima S. Aphasia and unilateral spatial neglect due to acute thalamic hemorrhage: clinical correlations and outcomes. *Neurological Sciences* 2016;37:565-572.

Otis JM, Zhu M, Namboodiri VMK, Cook CA, Kosyk O, Matan AM, Ying R, Hashikawa Y, Hasikawa K, Trujillo-Pisanty I, Guo J, Ung RL, Rodriguez-Rmaguera J, Anton E, Stuber GD. Paraventricular thalamus projection neurons integrate cortical and hypothalamic signals for cue-reward processing. *Neuron* 2019;103:423-431.

Parsons MP, Li S, Kirouac GJ. Functional and anatomic connection between the paraventricular nucleus of the thalamus and dopamine fibers of the nucleus accumbens. *Journal of Comparative Neurology* 2007;500:1050-1063.

Perry BAL and Mitchell AS. Considering the evidence for anterior and laterodorsal thalamic nuclei as higher order relays to cortex. *Frontiers in Molecular Neuroscience* 2019;12:[article]167, doi: 10.3389/fnmol.2019.00167[.]

Pettijohn KA and Radvansky GA. Walking through doorways causes forgetting: recall. *Memory* 2018;26:1430-1435.

Prasad JA, Carroll BJ, Sherman SM. Layer 5 corticofugal projections from diverse cortical areas: variations on a pattern of thalamic and extrathalamic targets. *Journal of Neuroscience* 2020;40:5785-5796.

Radvansky GA and Zacks JM. Event boundaries in memory and cognition. *Current Opinion in Behavioral Sciences* 2017;17:133-140.

Salazar-Juárez A, Escobar C, Aguilar-Roblero R. Anterior paraventricular nucleus modulates light-induced phase shifts in circadian rhythmicity in rats. *American Journal of Physiology Regulatory, Integrative and Comparative Physiology* 2002;283:R897-R904.

Schmahmann JD. Vascular syndromes of the thalamus. *Stroke* 2003;34:2264-2278.

Schulman S. Bilateral symmetrical degeneration of the thalamus; a clinicopathological study. *Journal of Neuropathology and Experimental Neurology* 1957;16:446-470.

Sebastian R, Schein MG, Davis C, Gomez Y, Newhart M, Oishi K, Hillis AE. Aphasia or neglect after thalamic stroke: the various ways they may be related to cortical hypoperfusion. *Frontiers in Neurology* 2014;5:article 231, published 19 November 2014, doi: 10.3389/fneur.2014.00231[.]

Sébille SB, Belaid H, Philippe A-C, André A, Lau B, François C, Karachi C, Bardinet E. Anatomical evidence for functional diversity in the mesencephalic locomotor region of primates. *NeuroImage* 2017;147:66-78.

Sherman SM. Functioning of circuits connecting thalamus and cortex. *Comprehensive Physiology* 2017;7:713-739.

Sherman SM and Guillery RW. The role of the thalamus in the flow of information to the cortex. *Philosophical Transactions of the Royal Society B* 2002;357:1695-1708.

Sherman SM and Guillery RW. Two types of thalamic relay: first order and higher order. In: *Exploring the Thalamus and Its Role in Cortical Function* [2nd ed.]. Cambridge and London: MIT Press, 2006a, pp. 290-316.

Sherman SM and Guillery RW. Function of burst and tonic response modes in the thalamocortical relay. In: *Exploring the Thalamus and Its Role in Cortical Function* [2nd ed.]. Cambridge and London: MIT Press, 2006b, pp. 290-316.

Sherman SM and Guillery RW. Thalamocortical links to the rest of the brain and the world. In: *Functional Connections of Cortical Areas. A New View from the Thalamus.* Cambridge and London: MIT Press, 2013a, pp. 217-244.

Sherman SM and Guillery RW. The dual nature of the thalamic input to cortex. In: *Functional Connections of Cortical Areas. A New View from the Thalamus.* Cambridge and London: MIT Press, 2013b, pp. 141-177.

Sherman SM and Koch C. Thalamus. In: *The Synaptic Organization of the Brain* [4th ed.]. New York and Oxford: Oxford University Press, 1998, pp. 221-251.

Smith Y, Raju D, Nanda B, Pare J-F, Galvan A, Wichmann T. The thalamostriatal systems: anatomical and functional organization in normal and parkinsonian states. *Brain Research Bulletin* 2009;78:60-68.

Stepniewska I, Preuss TM, Kaas JH. Thalamic connections of the dorsal and ventral premotor areas in new world owl monkeys. *Neuroscience* 2007;147:727-745.

Stern K. Severe dementia associated with bilateral symmetrical degeneration of the thalamus. *Brain* 1939;62:157-171.

Tanibuchi I and Goldman-Rakic PS. Dissociation of spatial-, object-, and sound-coding neurons in the mediodorsal nucleus of the primate thalamus. *Journal of Neurophysiology* 2003;89:1067-1077.

Thompson AN and Radvansky GA. Event boundaries and anaphoric reference. *Psychonomic Bulletin and Review* 2016;23:849-856.

Thompson SM and Robertson RT. Organization of subcortical pathways for sensory projections to the limbic cortex I. Subcortical projections to the medial limbic cortex in the rat. *Journal of Comparative Neurology* 1987;265:175-188.

Tierney AJ. Egas Moniz and the origins of psychosurgery: a review commemorating the 50th anniversary of Moniz's Nobel Prize. *Journal of the History of the Neurosciences* 2000;9:22-36.

Tokgoz S, Demirkaya S, Bek S, Kasikci T, Odabasi Z, Genc G, Yucel M. Clinical properties of regional thalamic hemorrhages. *Journal of Stroke and Cerebrovascular Diseases* 2013;22:1006-1012.

Van der Werf YD, Witter MP, Uylings HBM, Jolles J. Neuropsychology of infarctions in the thalamus: a review. *Neuropsychologia* 2000;38:613-627.

Van der Werf YD, Witter MP, Groenewegen HJ. The intralaminar and midline nuclei of the thalamus. Anatomical and functional evidence for participation in processes of arousal and awareness. *Brain Research Reviews* 2002;39:107-140.

Van Essen C. Visual areas of the mammalian cerebral cortex. *Annual Review of Neuroscience* 1979;2:227-263.

Vertes RP, Linley SB, Hoover WB. Limbic circuitry of the midline thalamus. *Neuroscience and Biobehavioral Reviews* 2015;54:89-107.

Von Holst E and Mittelstaedt H. *Das reafferens princip. Die Naturwissenschaften* 1950;37:464-476 [translated from the German in Dodwell F.C. [ed.]. *Perceptual Processing: Stimulus Equivalence and Pattern Recognition.* New York: Appleton Century Crofts, 1971].

Walshe TM, Davis KR, Fisher CM. Thalamic hemorrhage: a computed tomographic-clinical correlation. *Neurology* 1977;27:217-222.

Zachs JM and Tversky B. Event structure in perception and conception. *Psychological Bulletin* 2001;127:3-21.

Zhang D, Snyder AZ, Shimony JS, Fox MD, Raichle ME. Noninvasive functional and structural connectivity mapping of the human thalamocortical system. *Cerebral Cortex* 2010;20:1187-1194.

Zhou H, Schafer RJ, Desimone R. Pulvinar-cortex interactions in vision and attention. *Neuron* 2016;89:209-220.

www.ingramcontent.com/pod-product-compliance
Lightning Source LLC
Chambersburg PA
CBHW030745200526
45160CB00010B/65/J